MORE ADVANCED PRAISE FOR
ONE TICK STOPPED THE CLOCK

In *One Tick Stopped the Clock*, Jennifer Crystal courageously shares her journey through chronic illnesses, including Epstein Barr virus, multiple tick-borne diseases, and the challenges of being a long-hauler of COVID-19. With raw honesty and vulnerability, Jennifer sheds light on the struggles of seeking validation and understanding in a world where complex health conditions are often misunderstood. This memoir is a powerful testament to resilience, advocacy, and the unwavering spirit of those who continue to fight for recognition and empathy in the face of chronic illness.
—Laura M. MacNeill, M.B.A., CEO of Global Lyme Alliance

One Tick Stopped the Clock is a deeply moving journey of illness and redemption. Jennifer Crystal writes with clarity and insight, offering an essential read not just for anyone struggling with Lyme disease and its co-infections, but for the millions of people living with chronic illnesses who have had to overcome doubt and dismissal to find healing. Hers is an engaging and wise voice that brings to light the experiences of so many who remain unheard and unseen.
—Laurie Edwards, M.F.A., author of *Life Disrupted* and *In the Kingdom of the Sick*

One Tick Stopped the Clock is a cautionary tale of what could go wrong in modern medicine. Jennifer Crystal demonstrates how patients must often be proactive to be heard and healed, particularly when cases don't fit into a neat diagnostic box. Jennifer's story is, ultimately, a celebration of collaborative care that will serve as inspiration, both to patients seeking answers and to providers helping their patients achieve optimal health.
—Leana Wen, M.D., author of *When Doctors Don't Listen* and *Lifelines*

Jennifer Crystal is a beautiful writer, and she employs her simple yet lyrical prose to chronicle, through her individual story, the journey of long Lyme and tick-borne disease patients, writ large. From her eight years of misdiagnosis to her remission to searing relapse to a newfound balance, she journeys through the kingdom of the sick and emerges with the wisdom to seize life, nonetheless. This deeply felt narrative of illness and redemption offers an insider's understanding of the chronic Lyme journey and clear explanations of what such patients need to know to navigate the minefield themselves. Many patients have written books about their struggles with Lyme disease, but if you read just one—read this.

—Pamela Weintraub, author of *Cure Unknown* and senior editor at Aeon

Jennifer Crystal's story brings to light the often invisible world of chronic illness, drawing back the curtain on the lived patient experience. She showcases the damage that can be done when doctors don't take a proper history and carefully listen to a patient's narrative, and the health that can be restored when they do.

—Richard I. Horowitz, M.D., author of *Why Can't I Get Better? Solving the Mystery of Lyme & Chronic Disease* and *How Can I Get Better? An Action Plan for Treating Resistant Lyme & Chronic Disease*

Jennifer Crystal's story of mismanaged Lyme disease is infuriating, poignant, and all too common. Denial and ignorance thwarted her at every turn. When medicine could not offer help, it framed her symptoms as psychosomatic. Tick-borne illness afflicts more than a half million people yearly. Tests and treatments are known to fail often. And yet—at the doctor-patient level—people like Jennifer are dismissed, their pain manifestly compounded. Bravo for telling this wrenching story so well and in a way that supports tens of thousands of Lyme patients.

—Mary Beth Pfeiffer, Investigative Journalist, author of *Lyme: The First Epidemic of Climate Change*

In *One Tick Stopped the Clock*, Jennifer Crystal invites us into her ongoing story of navigating tick-borne illness and other chronic health conditions that are poorly understood and therefore often dismissed by the healthcare establishment. Her moving and achingly honest account sheds light on the frustration, invalidation, and exhaustion that so many patients face when their symptoms don't fit neatly into diagnostic algorithms and are ignored, or worse, chalked up to being "all in your head." Her story is a reminder to all patients to trust themselves and speak out, and a reminder to medical providers to listen well and never stop learning.

—Annie Brewster, M.D., Founder and Executive Director, Health Story Collaborative; Assistant Professor, Harvard Medical School; author of *The Healing Power of Storytelling*

A heartfelt memoir of one woman's courageous, convoluted, and ultimately redeeming journey through chronic illness.

—Steven Phillips, M.D., best-selling co-author of *Chronic: The Hidden Cause of the Autoimmune Pandemic and How to Get Healthy Again*

Anyone seeking to unravel the mystery of chronic illness should read this book. With raw honesty and vulnerability, Jennifer Crystal paints an intimate portrait of the physical, emotional, and mental challenges she faced every day. Readers are not only given a glimpse into the depths of her struggles, but also witness the incredible resilience and unwavering determination that propels her forward. This book is a beacon of hope. Prepare to be inspired, moved, and educated by this beautiful memoir.

—Dana Parish, best-selling co-author of *Chronic: The Hidden Cause of the Autoimmune Pandemic and How to Get Healthy Again*

Jennifer Crystal is an exceptional writer, a grand storyteller, sharing her personal, and sometimes horrific experience through the land of medical misdiagnosis, missed diagnoses, missed treatment opportunities and more during her chronic Lyme journey toward wellness. The reader is invited to join her in trying to solve the mysterious symptoms that it took eight long years to uncover. We feel the same sinking feeling in our stomachs when she realizes she will never return to who she was before tick-borne illness, in effect, life interrupted. Yet, like so much of our human story, she finds a way to not only survive, to continue, but to thrive, despite chronic illness. Hers is a story for our times—and beyond. As a colleague also with chronic illness notes in the book, "Your story is not just for Lyme patients. Anyone who's experienced trauma can learn from it." So can you.

—Ed O'Malley, Ph.D., Fellow, American Academy of Sleep Medicine

Jennifer Crystal explores the dysfunction of the medical system in dealing with those living with chronic illness—the blaming, the gaslighting, the denial. Her inspirational story offers hope to those looking to redefine their lives after a long illness.

—Kris Newby, author of *Bitten* and senior producer of *Under Our Skin*

Jennifer Crystal relates eloquently and with disarming forthrightness her decades-long descent into and eventual recovery from complex tick-borne illness. Her memoir demonstrates that with determination, an alliance with an equally determined health care practitioner and the support of family and friends, it is possible to regain relative wellness and lead a meaningful, successful, and happy life. Like others before her, such as Polly Murray and Ally Hilfiger, her inspiring and beautifully written work illuminates a path that others can follow.

—Kenneth B. Liegner, M.D., author of *Coping with Lyme Disease: A Practical Guide to Dealing with Diagnosis and Treatment*

One Tick Stopped the Clock powerfully illustrates how Lyme disease can derail a person's life, as well as the herculean effort it takes to get back on track. At 25, Jennifer Crystal had just snagged her dream job as a ski instructor, when out of the blue, her health went downhill fast. Unable to manage on her own, she landed back in her childhood bedroom, feeling hopeless and broken. This beautifully written memoir chronicles how she ultimately regained her health—no mean feat in a world that typically denies the

reality of "long-haul" Lyme disease—and found new dreams to replace those previously ripped away from her. An informative and inspiring read.
—Dorothy Kupcha Leland, President of LymeDisease.org, co-author of *When Your Child Has Lyme Disease: A Parent's Survival Guide* and *Finding Resilience: A Teen's Journey Through Lyme Disease*

Jennifer Crystal's meticulously detailed journey of her Lyme disease depicts the stories within the story of malpractice, prejudice, and ignorance visited upon long-haul patients by the disease care establishment, friends, and even family. Jennifer's heroic struggles, and the emergence of exceptional people, will inspire and guide many in the ME/CFS, EBV, and now long COVID communities.
—Alan Bachers, Ph.D., Director, Neurofeedback Foundation

A riveting story of a gifted young woman sinking into a chronic disabling illness. Jennifer's path to recovery and return to work as a writer are heartwarming.
—Daniel Cameron, M.D., author of *Inside Lyme*

Jennifer was a patient of mine for the better part of 15 years. Her dedication to the field, her time allotted to her own titanic struggle, and her ultimate success are all documented in her book. It is a moving story of one woman's grit and resolve in battling this insidious illness. Jennifer is an erudite and interesting writer as she narrates her personal struggle with this illness. She has also devoted a significant amount of time and energy in being a force in the Lyme community network. This book stands out as a testament to Jennifer's persistence and courage in her struggle to overcome the forces both personal and medical that were aligned against her. For those interested in this field this is a must-read memoir. Knowing Jennifer personally after these many years I am proud to acknowledge a supportive role in her return to health under normal daily life. This is a remarkable book and should be read by anyone interested in knowing more about tick-borne disease and its effect on the individual.

—Bernard Raxlen, M.D., author of *Lyme Disease: Medical Myopia and the Hidden Global Pandemic*

ONE TICK STOPPED THE CLOCK

a memoir

JENNIFER CRYSTAL

Legacy Book Press LLC
Camanche, Iowa

ISBN: 979-8-9891170-2-4
Library of Congress Case Number: 1-14058757971

AUTHOR'S NOTE

The events in this memoir are based on my own memories, as well as conversations with people involved, journal entries, medical files, emails, and notes. Opinions are my own, as is the story I tell; someone in the narrative might have different memories or feelings about shared experiences. Some names and identifying details have been changed to protect privacy, while others have been purposefully not changed per the person's request. Scientific information is either presented as it was explained to me by a medical professional, or it is cited. Certain excerpts or similar versions of anecdotes described here have been previously mentioned in blog posts for Global Lyme Alliance and lymedisease.org. Ten percent of the royalties earned from sales of this book will be donated to Global Lyme Alliance.

For the patients who need to be heard.
I believe you.

INTRODUCTION

When I started writing this book, the world had never heard of COVID-19. Words like "long hauler" and "immuno-compromised" were not part of the general lexicon. Those living in "the kingdom of the well," as author Susan Sontag once put it, had never experienced quarantine.

The other half, those living in "the kingdom of the sick,"[i] had long been halted due to illness. They were all too familiar with persistent symptoms that were often dismissed as psychosomatic. They knew what it was like for an illness to affect individuals differently, and for it to sometimes drag on longer than it was "supposed" to, with researchers debating why.

Over time, research and understanding of conditions like Myalgic Encephalomyelitis/Chronic Fatigue Syndrome (ME/CFS), fibromyalgia, Epstein-Barr virus, and Lyme disease have improved somewhat, but too many patients with illnesses that don't fit into simple diagnostic and treatment boxes are still unheard. Literacy is growing but often echoes in the chambers of the ill. Despite 476,000 new cases of Lyme disease in the U.S. each year—more than HIV and breast cancer combined[ii]—many people still don't understand the nuances of tick-borne disease, at least not beyond its early, acute manifestations. And that number pales in comparison to the 50 million Americans suffering from autoimmune diseases.[iii] These people either sink into an isolated

---

i   Sontag, Susan. *Illness as Metaphor.* New York: Vintage Books, 1977 (3).
ii   www.globallymealliance.org
iii   https://autoimmune.org/wp-content/uploads/2019/12/1-in-5-Brochure.pdf

existence of perpetual illness, or struggle to keep up with daily life while worrying that a flare-up could send them back to "lock-down" at a moment's notice.

In January 2021, *The New York Times Magazine* published an article titled "What if You Never Get Better From Covid-19?"[iv] Fellow Lyme disease patients sent it to me in frustration. "We haven't gotten better either," they exclaimed. "We have similar symptoms. Why is everyone talking about COVID long haulers when we've been suffering for years?"

As a long hauler of both COVID-19 and tick-borne disease, I understand that frustration. I also think it's precisely this attention on long-haul COVID that may finally shed light on—and bring credibility to—other persistent, complex illnesses.

For years before I was diagnosed with chronic Epstein Barr virus and multiple tick-borne illnesses, I fought just for people to believe that I was sick. Then, once I was properly diagnosed, I fought for understanding from people who did not believe in my diagnosis—as if a documented physical disease is simply an opinion or mystical power one can choose to believe in or not. Conversely, when I developed COVID-19 symptoms in March 2020, no one questioned whether I actually had the virus, despite a (false) negative test. No one said, "Oh, you must have something else" or, "It must just all be in your head." They knew my shortness of breath, dry cough, low-grade fever, and loss of taste and smell unequivocally meant COVID-19. When the positive antibody test came back that June, it was simply confirmation of what my doctors, friends, and family already knew to be true.

For the four months that I had acute COVID-19 and in the years that I've wrestled residual symptoms, I have only had to fight to get well, not to be believed. What a difference this validation has made! But I've been one of the lucky ones. Many COVID long haulers experience the dismissal that other chronic illness patients have suffered for years. The voices of those who don't fit a cookie-cutter medical mold, who have been sidelined, categorized, mislabeled, or hushed deserve to be heard. It's especially important to elevate the narratives of illnesses that are not in the forefront of the news, conditions that were around for years before the pandemic and will be for years to come. Illnesses that have no vaccines or herd

---

iv   https://www.nytimes.com/2021/01/21/magazine/covid-aftereffects.html

immunity. Illnesses that, like HIV/AIDS before them, are steeped in misunderstanding and controversy. Illnesses against which, like COVID-19, we can take preventive measures, but to which we are all still prone.

This is my story.

PART I

PROLOGUE

1997

My sandals squeaked in the soft sand as I made my way across the beach toward the water-skiing cove. Water-skiing was my favorite activity at the Maine sleepaway camp I attended as a camper and a counselor for ten summers. As a child, I raced across the beach to be the first to pick out skis and a lifejacket. As a nineteen-year-old counselor charged with driving the ski boat, I walked quickly and purposefully, knowing I had less than an hour to safely pull five campers around our area of the lake. I passed the canoeing, swimming, and sailing areas, walking about an eighth of a mile to the end of the sandy shore. A group of campers was already there, squabbling over equipment. When they saw me coming, they dropped the skis in the sand, shouting, "Can I go first? Can I go first?"

"You ladies work out the order while I get the boat," I instructed. "And remember…"

"…Not even your pinkie toe in the water until another counselor gets here," they chorused.

The camp's Boston Whaler, already worn and loved when I'd learned to ski behind it at age eleven, was moored at a dock 150 yards offshore. To get to it, I had to walk along a path in the woods that ran perpendicular to the shore. The water-skiing area marked a distinct line between the sunny, sandy beach and the shaded woods.

I never wore bug spray at camp. I spent all my time on or in the lake, so I thought I was immune to the bugs that hovered around

3

land activities. The only insects I worried about were mosquitoes, and they left with the humidity at the beginning of the summer. I was only concerned with dangers I could see. Besides minor scratches and the occasional stubbed toe, I didn't think about the implications of walking the ski boat path several times a day. It didn't occur to me that the woods were a thick nesting ground for animals and the bugs they host.

After a few minutes walking through brush and leaves that tickled my legs, I reached the dock. My sandals slapped against the faded boards, and I could hear the water lapping gently underneath. I waved at the campers back on shore, then knelt to undo the cleat knot that tied the boat to the dock. I unwound the faded yellow rope, twisting it around my hand as I leapt from the dock to the boat's bow. I walked to the stern to check the gas tanks. Satisfied, I sat down on the old wooden bench behind the steering wheel and turned the key. The boat roared to life. I heard the familiar *beep-beep* that meant everything was in working order.

"That's the sound I like to hear!" I said as I put the throttle in reverse and carefully maneuvered the boat away from the dock, turning toward the wider part of the lake to make a couple test runs. I revved the boat as if I were pulling a skier, a motion I could have done in my sleep. I loved that time alone in the boat, the wind whipping through my ponytail as I gunned the engine, the sun warming my face. As I slowed the boat to a stop, I closed my eyes for just a second, relishing the moment of stillness. I was totally in my element, tanned and healthy, filled with energy and the invincibility of youth.

As I opened my eyes and turned the boat, I happened to glance down at my right arm as it guided the steering wheel. Splattered across my forearm was a blotchy red rash. I stopped the boat and peered closer. The rash was a series of red dots that ran from my wrist halfway to my elbow. Past my outstretched arm, I could see the campers on shore, jumping up and down and waving to me to come get them already. I restarted the boat, deciding to focus on the task at hand and show the rash to the camp nurse later.

"Does it itch?" she asked when I presented it to her at lunch time.

"No."

The nurse that summer was from England, an R.N. who had treated patients on two continents. She was well-versed in the basic first aid issues that often arose at camp, but not aware of problems more endemic to the area, which at the time weren't high on anyone's radar. She ran her fingers over the rash. "It's not raised or anything. Does it hurt?"

"No."

"Well then, I wouldn't worry about it. We're at camp. It's probably from your sleeping bag or something. Let's just watch it for a few days and see what happens."

A few days later the rash faded. I didn't give it another thought.

CHAPTER 1

2003

The warm Colorado sun kissed my cheeks as my boyfriend Jim and I loaded onto a chairlift. I raised my goggles and closed my eyes, tilting my face toward the rays. "Nothing like a suntan in February."

The chairlift rose over a back bowl, a wide, open area where ski trails are so spacious that they're really just suggested "zones." The skiers below our lift were specks on a canvas of white that stretched for miles in every direction.

"Can't beat that Colorado blue sky either," Jim replied.

"Seriously, there should be a crayon called Ski Sky Blue."

The sky was the piercing cerulean of flawless Murano glass, unmarred by a single cloud. I thought of my friends back East, waking up to New York smog, or shivering against biting New England cold. I took a deep breath and smiled.

I'd always felt I could breathe easier in Rocky Mountain air, despite its high altitude. Growing up in Connecticut, I'd ski instructed locally on weekends in high school and had skied out West on family vacations. I couldn't wait to move to Colorado after college to spend a winter ski instructing in the Rockies.

I graduated from college on skis. Actually, to be fair, I was in a sled pulled by a ski patroller; the rest of my class was on skis, but we all came down the mountain in caps and gowns to celebrate our 2001 mid-year commencement in Vermont. A sign waiting at the bottom read: "Some were born to walk. Others were born to ski."

I was on crutches with crampons attached to the bottoms so I wouldn't slip on the snow and ice. Just a few weeks earlier, while interviewing for a ski instructing position out West, I'd torn the anterior cruciate ligament (ACL) in my left knee. Sailing over a ridge at too high a speed, I'd landed in an unexpected mogul field. Moguls, also known as "the bumps," require a certain speed and finesse to conquer effectively. You have to start slowly, survey the field from the top, and pick a line of moguls to ski through. If you keep your ski tips pointed downhill, you can simply bounce off the sides of each bump, until you hit the last one in your line. It takes leg strength, good timing, and a real command of your equipment to successfully ski a whole mogul line.

The day of my interview, I never made it past the first bump. Wholly unprepared for what was waiting over that smooth ledge, I tried to skid to a stop when I saw the field below me, but it was too late. I crashed into the side of a mogul. My lower left leg slammed forward while my torso fell back, pulling my thigh with it. My knee could not sustain that kind of split and gave way with a sickening snap.

The injury put me out for the rest of the ski season and shattered my plans to ski instruct after graduation. I was set on moving to Colorado, though. I packed up my green Jeep, covered in stickers that read "Ski today, work tomorrow" and "Ski like a girl," and drove 1500 miles west. I cheered at the prospect of adventure and exploration when my beloved Rocky Mountains at last came into view. I decided to look for a job off the hill that would still allow me to be part of the ski culture I craved. Years of camp counseling, and a lifetime of listening to my mother and stepfather talk at the dinner table about lesson plans, pointed me toward teaching. I became a third-grade assistant teacher, and then high school English teacher in Boulder, finding great joy in creating lesson plans, re-discovering favorite books, and bonding with students.

When I wasn't teaching, I was working overtime on leg lifts and hamstring curls, on exercises with red elastic pulleys tied to the foot of my dresser, trying to get myself as strong as the skiers all around me. It took two years for my knee to heal. Eventually I was able to ski as hard as I once had, to bounce through mogul fields again, but it took much longer than expected.

As Jim and I rode the chairlift to the top of the bowl, I patted the trusty knee brace hidden under my ski pants. "Two years ago, I never could have imagined I'd be out here."

Jim was taking me to a part of the mountain I'd never explored, a backcountry area accessible only on foot. After dismounting the chairlift, we glided to the outer limits of the authorized ski area. Flat areas, either on the top of trails or connecting them, are technically called "catwalks," or "the flats" in skier lingo. It's important to skate as fast as possible, like a cross-country racer, to gain momentum when heading into the flats. If you don't have enough speed to make it all the way across, you risk slowing to a stop, and it's nearly impossible to regain forward motion from there. Then it's endless shuffling along, dragging yourself by your poles, trying to walk with big boards strapped to your feet.

Jim and I used our poles to get ourselves going faster, faster, faster. Some people curl into a tuck, hunching over like downhill racers to bomb across the flats, but I always preferred slipping into a steady glide. I pushed off on my left ski, glided as far as possible, pressed my poles into the snow to help me along, then pushed off on my right ski. Glide, pole, back to the left. As we skated across the ridge, I sensed that all at once everything was working in sync: my skis, my poles, the mountain, the air, my breathing.

I followed Jim along the catwalk, past the area where we'd spent countless hours tree skiing. We wove among groups of skiers trying to decide if they wanted to brave the trees, but the packs dwindled the farther we skated. Eventually it was just the two of us, gliding, poling, breathing. Without slowing my pace, I reached for the mouthpiece of the pack that carried water on my back. I was glad I had it to help keep me going. I also wondered what would happen if—when—I had to pee.

The flats thinned as we passed the last bowl. "This looks good," I shouted. If we dropped down to our right, there was a whole area of fresh snow waiting for our tracks.

"Nah, keep going," Jim called back without turning his head. I took another long sip of water. I could already feel sweat pooling in my armpits. Finally, several minutes later, Jim skidded to a stop below a crag. Snow covered only part of the rocks, dripping over them like melted frosting. "We're here!" he announced triumphantly.

I opened the pit zips on my jacket. "You brought me all the way out here for rocks?"

"No, silly. This is where we climb"—Jim pointed above the crag, where I could just make out the glaring white of untouched powder—"to heaven on earth."

"Up over these rocks?"

"Up over these rocks. After that, it's just straight uphill on snow. If we stick by those trees up there, the snow will be more packed, and it'll be easier to walk." Jim pointed to the few scraggly evergreens that had managed to survive at 11,000 feet.

I gulped. Nevertheless, when Jim crouched down, I reluctantly straddled his shoulders. He straightened, lifted me by the underside of my thighs like an ice skater, and hoisted me up so that I was essentially hugging the base of the crag. I felt my left boot *thunk* hard on Jim's arm as I tried to swing my legs toward the rock. "Sorry, sorry!"

"You're good." He held me as I worked to steady my boots. I engaged every muscle in my arms and legs to scurry up and over the crag, landing on top with a belly flop. The bottom of my jacket scrunched up around my bellybutton. Cold, wet slush pressed against my stomach. I turned my face to the side so as not to get a mouthful of snow.

"Nice!" Jim cheered. "Now scoot yourself around so you're facing me, and I'll hand you the gear."

Jim handed me our skis and poles. I planted everything in the snow so it would stay put and out of the way while Jim climbed up. He instructed me to lay flat on the top of the crag with my arms reaching out towards him. I was reminded of lifeguard training at summer camp, lying flat on a wooden dock to secure my own weight while pulling someone else to safety. I dug the front of my ski boots into the snow, just as I used to dig my feet into the dock, concentrating on keeping my weight on the bottom half of my body. I reached for Jim's hands. Grasping them, he planted his feet on the rock so fast that I was only carrying his full weight for a second. I placed his hands on the top of the snowy rock, my hands over them, just as I'd secured tired swimmers' hands on the dock.

"I've got it," he said. "You can let go."

I pulled my hands away and scooched backwards to give Jim room to land. As soon as he did, he clapped his gloves together. "Okay, let's hike up! I'll carry the skis. You take the poles."

Slowly we made our way up the hill, keeping close to the trees, which grew sparser the higher we climbed. The ascent was akin to walking up a sledding hill, though the climb was much higher and sweatier. I kept the water backpack mouthpiece between my lips, so that my pace became *huff, puff*, gulp, step. At last, we reached the summit. Jim placed our skis in the snow, and I planted our poles next to them. We sat down with a gentle thump. The powder cushioned me like a fluffy cotton pillow.

"Feel how soft it is?" Jim asked. "This snow has been piling up all season, just waiting for us." We were above tree line, the only living things in a sea of white that glowed against the intense blue sky. "Just think," Jim added, "Next winter we'll be able to come out here all the time!"

I had decided not to renew my teaching contract for the following school year, so that I could finally fulfill my lifelong dream of ski instructing for a season. I loved teaching, but I felt I was living on the periphery of the life I had truly sought out West. My students couldn't understand why I was leaving them. For weeks I'd vacillated about the decision, feeling like a mother who was about to abandon her children. I wasn't ready to be a mother, though, certainly not literally but not really even figuratively. I'd moved 1500 miles away from home to do what I loved to do: ski. Time seemed to be running short to fulfill that dream. I thought, *It's not like I can drop everything and become a ski bum ten years from now, wherever I might be, probably working and married with kids.*

Jim was also a teacher, in a town closer to the mountains. We'd met on a chairlift. A friend and I were gliding into a quadruple chairlift line when a tall, broad-shouldered guy slid in next to us. "Single?" he'd asked. This is the term skiers use when they're wondering if you have a single spot open in your group to share a chair ride.

I was feeling sassy that day, high from an exhilarating morning on the slopes, so I'd replied, "Why yes, actually, I am."

Jim had skied with us that whole morning, and then asked for my phone number. I never thought he'd call, but he did, the very next day, and before I knew it, the random guy I'd met on the chairlift had become my boyfriend. While he wasn't the reason I was moving to the mountains, being geographically closer to him was going to be a bonus. We each planned to spend one more year in Colorado. I had a dream of someday becoming a professor, and I hoped that after our final ski season out West, Jim and I would make the leap to graduate school together.

I scanned the glistening panorama below us and turned to Jim. "You're right, this is heaven on earth."

He shook his head and jumped to his feet. "Not quite yet." He clicked into his skis. I stood up to put mine on too, holding onto Jim for balance. Once we were ready, we grabbed our poles and pushed off straight across the top of the hill. Suddenly, Jim dropped down to his right and made a wide, arcing turn. "This is it!" he shouted. "Drop in! Don't use your poles. Just lean back and enjoy the ride!"

Nervously, I pointed my skis downhill. I'd never been in powder that deep, and I wasn't sure I knew how to ski it. Back East, I'd learned to lean as far forward as possible, carving sharp turns on the edges of my skis. Days of soft powder in the Rockies had reversed that thinking, teaching me to lean back and let the snow guide me, but it had never been so deep or soft that I hadn't needed my poles to help carve turns.

I pushed off and immediately started giggling. I was afraid I'd sink in all that powder, but my skis just glided right through it like I was skiing in a cloud. I attempted to carve a turn but realized that wasn't necessary. All I had to do was lean a little bit in one direction or the other, and my skis simply drifted. My poles dangled at my sides.

"This is so cool!" I squealed. "I'm floating! No, I'm FLYING!" I shouted and laughed all the way down, wishing the ride would never end.

If I had known how quickly it would, I might have insisted that the hands of time be stopped.

CHAPTER 2

Three months later, I wearily pulled into a motor lodge somewhere in Pennsylvania. I don't remember the name of the motel, or the town in Pennsylvania it was in. It was supposed to be a forgotten resting point, not the place where my quarter-life crisis would officially begin. I'd been driving for three days. After finishing the school year, I was heading to Maine for my tenth summer at camp, now as a Head Counselor and water-skiing director. I'd spend the summer there and then return to Colorado to ski instruct for the winter. I was supposed to make the cross-country trek with Jim. Instead, I'd driven straight across the Midwest by myself, accompanied only by swaying corn fields, enormous freight trucks that made my Jeep look like an ant, and the occasional cow on the side of the road. Finally, I pulled into the motel parking lot and stumbled into the main office to book a room.

On my twenty-fifth birthday in early May, Jim and I had toasted "To us!" Days later, he'd suddenly announced his "feelings had changed." No amount of arguing or protesting could get him to explain or reconsider. Just when I thought we were getting more serious, he walked out of my life as quickly as he'd skied into it.

"He's a schmuck," my hometown best friend Sharon told me over the phone as I lugged my bags into the motel room in Pennsylvania, grumbling to her about the recent breakup. "He doesn't deserve you."

Cradling the phone with my chin so I could use both hands to double lock the door, I said, "I get that, rationally. I just never expected this to happen. This wasn't part of the plan."

"But you're still going to spend a season in the mountains," Sharon reminded me. "That's been your dream since we were kids and you're about to live it. You don't need him."

I dropped my keys on the bureau and sat down on the bed. The room was dusty and dark, with heavy maroon curtains that matched the worn bedspread. The stagnant air was thick with stale air freshener, the carpeting so dank that I kept my flip flops on.

"You're a strong person," Sharon said. "You always come out the other side, just like with your knee. You'll be at camp soon, and this will all be behind you."

I felt better for a moment, picturing the camp's crystal-clear lake that had welcomed me home for ten summers. I couldn't wait to be nestled among the pines on the shore, laughing with friends I'd known since we were campers ourselves.

Despite the happy visual, I was suddenly overcome with fatigue. Laying back on the thin pillows, I muttered to Sharon, "Thanks for talking. I'm going to rest for a bit." I hung up and closed my eyes.

Bouts of low energy were not unusual for me. Like most twenty-somethings, I often sacrificed sleep for the sake of spending time with friends, hitting the slopes, or staying up until the wee hours grading papers. I seemed to get sick more often than my peers, but my body was young, and I could generally count on it to rebound when I pushed it too hard. Whenever sleep pleaded with me, I simply ignored it and relied on adrenaline to kick in and keep me going.

What was alarming that night in Pennsylvania was that nothing kicked in. It was as if someone had hit the off button and my whole system shut down. I lay in the darkening room, sensing the sun setting outside the thick curtains. After an hour or so, my stomach grumbled, but I couldn't bring myself to get up. I fumbled for the phone on the nightstand and ordered a heaping plate of undercooked, overpriced room service pasta. I ate it in bed, staring at cheap paintings of mountains, the standard artwork of motel rooms across America.

After dinner, I changed into a pair of raggedy boxer shorts and a tee shirt and climbed into bed for real. When I was driving that day, I'd promised myself I'd go for a run around the motel parking lot the next morning, since I felt like a slug from sitting in the car for so long. As I set my alarm, however, I wasn't even sure I'd be able to get up at 7:00 a.m. I set the alarm for 10:00 a.m. Then I turned out the light.

But I didn't fall asleep. As I closed my eyes, I felt the familiar sensation of a low blood sugar reaction coming on. Even though I'd just eaten, I was once again starving, the hunger gnawing like a hollow space that ran from the center of my head to the pit of my stomach. "I just finished a huge dinner," I groaned aloud. "Can't I please sleep?" My body ignored my plea, responding instead with a racing heart, sweaty palms, and a dizziness that would have made me pass out had I not been lying down.

These blood sugar crashes had been coming on at nonsensical times for six years. The first occurred at camp in 1997, the same summer I'd found the strange red rash on my arm. I had just walked into the dining hall for lunch. The room held rows of long wooden tables and benches. As I sat down at the head of a table in the center row, the room started spinning. Everything became blurry. I could hear the din of the campers but couldn't make out what they were saying. Through hazy vision I discerned their worried faces. Quickly, I rose from the table, and just as quickly, my gelatin knees gave out.

With the help of the camp nurse, I made my way to the adjacent counselor's room and sank down on a tattered couch. My heart raced. With clammy hands, I tried to wipe the sweat off my brow. Black splotches danced menacingly in front of my eyes. As the room started to grow dark, the nurse put a dry plastic spoon in my mouth. I tasted the succulent juice of perfectly ripened blueberries mixed with sweet syrup.

Within moments, the shaking subsided. Sensation returned to my lips, my cheeks, and finally my appendages. Everything in the room started to come into focus; blurred images morphed back into smiling faces and concerned eyes.

The nurse propped my head on a pillow and handed me a glass of orange juice and some crackers with peanut butter. "You had a low blood sugar reaction," she said. "You should get tested for diabetes."

Tests later showed I was not diabetic, but I was hypoglycemic, a condition I'd never heard of before that summer. I learned if a person with hypoglycemia doesn't eat at regular intervals, their blood sugar can drop dangerously below 70 milligrams per deciliter of blood, causing the symptoms I experienced.[i] I didn't understand why I would suddenly develop this condition at camp, where I ate well and took better care of my body than I did the rest of the year. No one seemed too concerned with the answer. I was told to simply keep little snacks on hand, and to make sure I ate regular meals.

The low blood sugar reaction I experienced in the Pennsylvania motel room, six years after the first one in 1997, was similar to the crashes I'd felt so many times before. I got out of bed and shuffled in the dark to reach my bags, scrounging up a package of cookies from the bottom of my purse. I ate them quickly, not even bothering to get a glass of water to wash them down, and got back into bed. Within minutes I felt better and finally drifted into a deep sleep.

When the alarm went off the next morning, I felt like I'd been sleeping for only an hour, two at most. But when I peeked out from under the covers, I saw that the clock glowed 10:03. I rubbed my eyes. My body felt like lead.

I would have drifted right back to sleep, had I not happened to swallow as I turned my head against the pillow. The pain in my throat suddenly had me wide awake. I sat up and swallowed again. *Maybe I was just lying in a funny position,* I thought. *Maybe there are still pieces of cookie stuck in my throat.* I swallowed a few more times. No, it was definitely a sore throat. Instinctively, I reached up and felt the sides of my neck; my glands were swollen, too. *Great. Now what?* I needed to get to Connecticut to visit with my family before I was due to arrive at camp in less than a week. I didn't have time to be sick.

I plodded to the bathroom. My face was pale, the skin around my brown eyes puffy and framed with dark circles. I splashed cold water on my face. *You're sick. Just get back into bed, sleep,*

---

i https://www.cdc.gov/diabetes/basics/low-blood-sugar.html

and drive tomorrow. The rational side of me contemplated this idea for about three seconds. Then the go-go-go, do-do-do side of me took over, as it always did, and tucked prudence under the covers without me.

I threw on a cotton sundress, gathered my long dark hair into a messy bun, and hit the road before I could rethink my plan. I drove with all the windows open and the music blaring, sucking on a lollipop as a sort of two-in-one remedy for my throbbing throat and mounting fatigue. This worked until halfway across the New Jersey turnpike, when exhaustion threatened to take over the way it had the night before.

It was 2:30 in the afternoon. Undoubtedly, I had a fever. *But you're just a few hours from Connecticut. You can't stop now.* I did permit myself to stop at a rest area, but instead of using the place for reasons its name would suggest, I simply bought some fake energy in the form of a soda and a chocolate ice cream cone.

When I at last trudged up the stone walkway to my mother and stepfather's house, I was bordering on delirium.

"Jen's home!" my mom called out as she pushed open the screen door to greet me.

"I don't feel so good," I whimpered, giving her a limp hug.

"You don't look so good." My mom smoothed her hand across my forehead. "You're warm."

I walked into the kitchen where my stepfather and fifteen-year-old half-sister Elizabeth were sitting at the round oak table. Elizabeth grimaced when she saw me; she was probably wondering if this is how breakups always made people look and was reconsidering her recent interest in boys.

"I made your favorite," my mother chirped. She put on her old green apron and collected the white plates off the table, loading them with sizzling stacks of eggplant parmesan. The food looked so good, but I was too tired to eat it. All I wanted to do was sleep. So just like in the *Peter Rabbit* stories she used to read me at bedtime, my mom replaced my dinner with chamomile tea and sent me to bed. We both figured a good night's sleep would do the trick.

My first thought when I awoke the next morning was, *There are needles in my throat.* Slowly, I sat up and got out of bed. My head was foggy. If there was any question left about calling a doctor, one glance in the bathroom mirror sealed the deal. My glands were enormous. I looked like one of those blown-up frogs on the cover of high school Biology books.

Having lived in Colorado for two years, I no longer had a doctor in Connecticut. I called my mother at work. "Who is this?" she asked when my voice came out in a husky rasp.

"It's me, Jen. Your daughter?"

"Oh, you sound awful." She gave me the number for a doctor she'd recently seen. "Don't worry," my mom said as we hung up. "You probably have strep. All you need is a few days of antibiotics and you'll be good to go."

The doctor was so sure of this same diagnosis that she didn't bother to do a strep culture when I saw her later that day. Handing me a prescription for a short course of antibiotics, she said, "You'll be fine in a few days."

A few days later, I was anything but fine. The glands on my neck had gotten larger, and others had painfully popped out all over my body. My sore throat, dotted each day with bigger and bigger white spots, only permitted me to eat soup, applesauce, and popsicles; in just three days, I'd dropped six pounds. Despite round-the-clock ibuprofen, a low-grade fever persisted. I slept more than twenty hours a day.

"You need to give the medicine time to work," the doctor said when I called to say my symptoms had only gotten worse.

"I thought antibiotics are supposed to kick in within forty-eight hours."

The doctor sighed. "That's true, but obviously you have a very bad case of strep, so it'll probably take longer."

I wasn't convinced. Taking a deep breath, I said what a part of me already knew was true but hadn't wanted to admit. "Do you think I might have mono?"

"There's no way you have mono," she replied. "You don't have any of the symptoms."

I furrowed my brow in confusion. I'd been tested for mono enough times in college to know the typical symptoms: sore throat, swollen glands, fever, and fatigue. Sophomore year, after the summer at camp when I found the rash and developed hypoglycemia, I'd been plagued by a flu that rendered me unable to attend class or even walk to the dining hall. When a mono test came back negative, I was told that I was probably just stressed or run down. That same flu came back on and off throughout college. Each time it did, I prayed that I didn't have mono; I knew how long it could take to get over that virus, and I didn't have time for it.

Even though previous mono tests had always come back negative, I had a bad feeling this time would be different; this felt worse than my usual flu. "I'd like to get tested anyway, just to be sure," I requested.

Over the few days as I waited for the test results, I talked myself out of my own reasoning and started to believe the doctor's words. When her nurse called, I greeted her cheerily, croaked, "Thanks!" and almost hung up before I heard her ask if I understood what she'd said. "It's positive. Your mono test was positive."

"What?!" I held the phone away from my face, grimacing at it as if it were the virus itself. Positive? *Positive?* "Are you sure?" My voice caught.

"Yes. I'm sorry. Be sure to get plenty of rest, and drink lots of fluids." The nurse didn't sound so sorry. She sounded like she was delivering the weather report, and if I'd please just thank her and hang up, she could move on to her next call.

"But…wait. I mean, is that really all I can do? How long will it take?"

"It's a virus. There's nothing you can do but rest. It usually takes about two weeks to get over the acute symptoms, maybe longer."

"Two weeks? I don't have two weeks!" My mind spun, thinking of the pre-camp training sessions I was supposed to run in less than forty-eight hours, of the counselors in my unit who would need a leader, of my campers who would look to me to comfort their homesickness in just a few nights. "You don't understand," I whined. "I *have* to be in Maine in two days."

"I'm sorry," the nurse said again. "But you have mono. You can't."

"Can't" was not part of my vocabulary. As a Taurus, my stubbornness didn't let me take "no" for an answer. There was no way I was letting what must have been a parting gift from Jim hold me back from a summer at camp, a tonic I needed more than ever.

I told the doctor as much when I went to her office later that day to see if there was anything she could tell me that the nurse on the phone hadn't. I'm not sure why I even went back to that doctor after she'd been wrong about mono, but I was desperate.

"Tell me exactly what you'd be doing at camp," she said as she felt my liver and spleen, organs that can become dangerously enlarged and possibly ruptured from mono.

I gave her a watered-down description of my responsibilities, stressing the time I'd spend just sitting in the ski boat and the rest hour and free periods built into the schedule when I could sleep. I neglected to mention that as a Head Counselor, my free time was often usurped by problems in my unit I needed to solve; that late-night meetings frequently kept me up well past "Taps"; that as the oldest returning counselor, the camp directors would count on my leadership in ways that didn't allow for a "step back and rest" attitude. But so narrow was my tunnel vision of getting to camp that even I seemed to have forgotten just how much energy my job required.

"Well, your liver and spleen are not enlarged," the doctor said tentatively, "but you're still very sick."

"What about steroids?" I'd read they could help alleviate the acute symptoms of mono.

The doctor pursed her chapped lips. "That's a very new technique. It's still controversial and is only used in very serious cases."

"Which mine is!"

The doctor tapped her pen on her notebook and her right navy ballet flat on the floor. "All right," she finally relented. "I'll give you the prescription."

I smiled for the first time in days.

"You still need to take it very, very easy," she cautioned as she handed me the coveted piece of white paper. "You can't go to camp until at least the Fourth of July."

That was just over two weeks away! The permission to still go to camp suddenly made a two-week delay seem not so bad at all.

Friends who'd had mono cautioned that the fatigue could last much longer than the prescribed two weeks and that going to camp would be too much of a push. My father expressed concern when I called to tell him my plan. "I'm worried you're going to wear yourself out and you won't be ready to ski this winter. You've got to think long-term."

"I can't miss camp," I insisted. "They've already got another Head Counselor starting late. They really need me there." My blinders didn't let me see that my seemingly selfless proffer of help was, in fact, quite selfish. What camp really needed was for me to give my all, and I wasn't going to be able to do that. I was also blinded by the young, naïve mentality that eventually, illness went away. I knew so few chronically ill people that I could express sympathy for them, but did not understand their lived experience, and certainly never thought it could happen to me. I was sick a lot, but I always got better. I thought resilience meant pushing through, not stopping to rest.

"I'll be fine by fall," I assured my dad. "Most people get over mono in a month. The steroids are going to make recovery go a lot faster."

"You're sure?" It was unlike my father to suggest I give something up; he always wanted me to keep going, to strive higher. The fact that he was so concerned about me going to camp should have been a warning of the serious jeopardy in which I was putting my future plans, but I simply said, "Winter is a long time away. I can always rest more in the fall if I need to. I'll be fine for ski season."

My mind was made up. I rested for two weeks, as promised. My acute symptoms cleared up. On July 5th, I got back in my Jeep and made the five-hour trip from Connecticut to Maine.

CHAPTER 3

"Okay ladies, let's line up by unit," I called out to the whole camp after our picnic supper on the night I arrived. It was council fire night, and one of my jobs was to lead the songs and organize the general operation of that weekly ritual. I watched as the girls raced to stand behind their counselors on the dirt path that led to the grassy area in front of the dining hall.

I walked toward the council fire tree. Thick and slightly bent, it had long supported the back of the counselor who led council fire; she stood against it as she sang the song that signaled the rest of camp to file in, past the tree into an inner and outer circle. I remember looking up at the counselor who played this role when I was a camper. Now, I was proud to stand in her place.

I glanced at the lake to my right. The sun was just starting to set, casting streams of pink that made the water shimmer. The water was completely still, except for a few small waves that lapped against the rocks by shore. It was a sound I'd known since childhood. Feeling totally centered, I took my place against the tree and looked back toward the campers and counselors. I started to sing, their cue to start walking. I loved seeing each smiling face as the girls went by. Some gave a little wave. One counselor scrunched her nose and raised her eyebrows up and down, trying to make me laugh. Another whispered, "Thank goodness you're here."

The exhilaration of being at camp and the false energy that carried over from the steroids at first made me think I was completely over mono. My head felt clear, I was excited to teach water sports, and I slept well at night. But that high quickly faded, and within a couple weeks it felt like I was dragging my body along with me to activities. I only taught three activities a day instead of four, which frustrated the camp director, Pam. She'd known I was going to have limitations but seeing them in practice was difficult for everyone involved. Even though I took on extra responsibility helping out in cabins that were having trouble, training new staff, taking the counselors water-skiing during free time, and generally lending an experienced hand to make sure camp ran smoothly, I got the sense Pam thought I was being lazy when I needed to rest. A former professional athlete, she was used to working with people who pushed their bodies beyond normal limits. My heart and mind wanted so badly to meet those expectations, but my body simply couldn't do it.

As the summer wore on, so did my energy. It wasn't the buzzy tiredness of staying up too late, the droopy-eyed fatigue of a long day of activity, or the sore muscle burn of a good workout. Sometimes I felt so exhausted that I wanted to cry, but I got up anyway to teach canoeing and swimming. I thought I was some kind of martyr, but in reality, there were no points to be earned, no prize to be won except the silver pendant of a water-skier that I received at the end of the summer to commemorate my ten years at camp.

Even though I knew I'd pushed my body too hard by going to camp, I still thought the mono would be gone by the end of the summer. I believed pushing myself was a good thing; I was sure I could get through anything with sheer determination. I saw my life playing out like a movie. No matter what happened, everything would eventually work out.

But everything was not okay when I parked my Jeep in front of my apartment in Boulder in late August. I planned to recuperate there for a few months before moving up to the mountains. Luckily, my camp friend Rachel had shared the cross-country drive with me this time. She ended up doing most of the driving. It felt weird to be a passenger in my own car.

As we approached Boulder, I took over once more; it seemed important for me to be in the driver's seat when I arrived home.

A few blocks from my apartment, Rachel asked if we could stop at a convenience store. I spotted one and turned in to its narrow parking lot, which had clearly been designed before the boom of ever-growing SUVs. As I edged the Jeep into a small space, I heard a sickening crunch on the left side of the car.

"What was that?!" Rachel exclaimed, wide-eyed.

Reluctantly, I put the car in park, opened my door, and stepped down to see that the entire driver's side was smushed in. The culprit was a bright yellow pole, just under my line of vision, which was meant to guide snowplows. "But it's summer! Why is this pole even here?" I kicked it and winced. The pole was cemented to the ground.

"It was in your blind spot," Rachel said as she, too, got out of the car and came around to survey the damage. "You couldn't have seen it." She traced her hands over the dent, trying to scrape off some of the yellow paint streaked across the Jeep. She opened and closed the doors. "Well, it's still drivable. The doors work. Let's just get settled in your apartment and you can deal with it later."

I don't remember what Rachel bought at the convenience store. I do remember how deflated I felt when we pulled up to my apartment. I was unusually lightheaded as I dragged a suitcase up the front walk. My body seemed to be gulping for air. I'd never had a problem with re-entry to high altitude before.

For the first few days back in Boulder, I spiked fevers. My joints ached. Rachel would go out for a few hours and walk around the city, but when she came back, I was no better. I felt bad that I couldn't be a good host, and finally called another camp friend Heather, who lived nearby, to come get Rachel.

Alone in my apartment, I agonized over how I would get well enough to move to the mountains as my symptoms persisted into early fall. I wished I'd listened to those who'd cautioned me not to go to camp. I'd lie in bed wondering, *Is my dream of ski instructing going to be thwarted by a medical issue once again?*

Night after night I stared at the ceiling. Eventually I'd doze off for a few fitful hours, but those were filled with crazy nightmares. I dreamed I was running away from a predator, fighting with someone, collapsing after being shot in the head, or getting stabbed in the heart. I survived in those dreams even when I shouldn't have, but I woke up shaken and more tired than I was when I went to sleep.

I didn't tell anyone about the nightmares because I assumed they were a reaction to my daytime worries. I didn't want people to think I was weak. If I could just get control of my emotions, of my health, I could make everything better.

"And you're feeling better?" my father asked every Sunday when I spoke to him and my stepmother Janet.

"Well, still tired," I replied each week.

"But you're noticing some improvement."

"I guess…" I wasn't really, but I didn't know what else to say.

"And you're still planning on moving to the mountains." No matter what negative scenario I'd ever described to him, from scraping my knee to losing a student council election, my father turned it around with a statement like, "But you're still…" I think it was his way of trying to put a positive spin on the narrative. I also know that he likes order and plans. I didn't want to make him nervous. I, too, wanted to believe that with just a few more weeks of rest, I would get well and move forward with my life dream.

Heather came to visit and saw first-hand how I was struggling. "It's Saturday, and I have to go food shopping, so I bet you do, too," she said. "Get a list together and I'll shop for you this afternoon." Some newer friends were not as understanding. One weekend, I scheduled lunch with my former teaching colleagues. I knew my energy would last longer if I didn't have to worry about driving, so I asked one of them if she could pick me up.

"I hate to say that's really going to be tough," she sighed into the phone. "I've got a lot to do this morning and it's going to take an extra ten minutes to swing by your apartment." I think in her mind, I was supposed to be over mono by now. Having not experienced anything like it herself, she may have seen my lingering fatigue, and my request, as laziness. Had I not been sick myself, I might have seen someone in my shoes the same way. Prolonged illness was not familiar for us, especially in a pre-COVID-19 world.

Eventually the truth about my nightmares leaked out to my mother. I called her one morning sobbing, "This guy was in the elevator with me with a torch. He set my hair on fire, and I was burning but couldn't move but was somehow still alive and," I heaved, "and this kid Jon that I knew in elementary school was there in the hallway, and the hallway became a cloud, and…"

"Whoa," my mom said. "Stop. It wasn't real. You're awake now. These dreams are crazy, though. You've never had dreams like this."

"I've never felt this sick. My whole body aches."

"Like aches when you get the flu?"

"Kind of. It feels like something is pulling on my muscles and joints and bones." There were other strange new symptoms, too. "I have these weird burning sensations in my hands and feet at night. About an hour after I get into bed, they start to get really hot. It feels like my blood is boiling, not like I'm getting warm from something external like a blanket."

"That's terrible," my mother tisked. "Maybe you should go see your doctor out there?"

"She'll tell me I have mono. I already know that."

"Maybe there's something else going on besides mono. I never had achiness or burning extremities when I had mono."

I'd visited my Colorado primary care doctor many times over the previous two years for sinus infections, ear infections, bronchitis, and migraines. She'd treated each symptom or infection separately, never questioning why I was sick so often, or what could be causing the headaches. I didn't expect her to have anything new to say about mono. Nevertheless, I scheduled an appointment and got a complete blood workup.

"Well, Crystal, your blood work shows that you still have mono," she said matter-of-factly as she walked into the exam room.

"Jennifer," I said.

"What?" The doctor sat down on a pink swivel stool.

"My name is Jennifer. My last name is Crystal. But it's okay, people get it mixed up all the time." By people I meant her; we'd been through this at least six or seven times.

"Oh…sorry." She flipped through my chart. Her blonde hair hung in front of her eyes, making it difficult to see her expression as she spoke. "Anyway, you've had mono long enough now that it's slipped into chronic Epstein-Barr virus."

"Isn't that the virus that causes mono?"

"Yes." The doctor swiveled to face me. "Everyone who tests positive for mono will test positive for EBV. But eventually, when the mono goes away, the EBV titers should decrease, showing evidence only of past infection. Yours are very high, meaning the infection is still active."

"So, what do I do?"

"There's not much you can do, I'm afraid." The doctor stuck her lower lip out. I focused on her shiny pink lip gloss; I wanted some just like it for nights out in the mountains. "The only cure is rest," she interrupted my thoughts. "Rest, rest, rest."

"I'm resting." For once, I could say that honestly.

"Good, then keep it up. It can take a very long time to get over EBV."

"What about the aches?" I shifted on the exam table. "And the burning sensations?"

"I'd take some ibuprofen for the aches. I'm not sure about the burning. I've never heard of that before. Let's just monitor it, and maybe you can see an infectious disease doctor if it doesn't get better." She snapped my chart closed and started to stand.

"Um…but…I'm supposed to ski instruct this winter." I grinned sheepishly.

The doctor sat back down. She pursed her pink lips, waited a moment to speak. "I don't know about that, Crystal."

"Jennifer."

"Yes, Jennifer. Sorry. Ski instructing takes a lot of energy. You're telling me you're in bed twenty hours a day. Are you really going to be ready to be on a mountain in just a couple of months? Even if you start to regain your strength, your muscles will be very weak."

This was not what I wanted to hear. I needed this doctor to tell me that another few weeks of rest would be ample time to get over mono, even if it was now EBV. Instead, she said, "It can take some people a year, maybe two, to get over EBV. The infection is chronic. Even if you start to feel better, it's always going to be in your system, and you're going to have to be really careful not to let it flare up. You're going to have to pace yourself. Your fatigue is going to stick around for a while. I can't imagine ski instructing would be a good idea."

I drew my hands over my face. I could not, would not believe that this dream was about to be shattered again. I had no contingency plan. "What would you do?" I asked the doctor.

"If I were you, I would call the mountain and tell them it's not going to work for this season."

"And then what?"

"Well, you're not teaching anymore, right?"

I shook my head.

"I'd stay with family for a while." She rotated again on her stool. "You're not well enough to work, and you need a place to just recuperate."

"My family lives in Connecticut," I told her.

"Do you have any other ties here in Colorado?"

I thought for a minute. Without a job, without a boyfriend, what was keeping me? "Friends," I replied. "And I love it here."

"Well, Colorado will be here. So will your friends. But you need to get well. If I were you, I'd go home."

As if it were that simple. Where was home?

CHAPTER 4

My parents divorced when I was a baby. My dad married my stepmom Janet when I was two, and my mom re-married when I was six. I grew up with my mom and stepdad just west of Hartford, Connecticut, and spent one weekend a month and some vacations with my dad and Janet in a Connecticut suburb of New York City. When I went away to college and then moved to Colorado, I went "home" to Connecticut to visit both families, but I had established myself elsewhere.

But now I couldn't fend for myself, and I couldn't stretch my camp salary long enough to keep paying my rent in Boulder. I wasn't functioning as an adult. I couldn't work, I couldn't cook, and I could barely stand long enough to bathe.

I was scared to tell my parents what the doctor had recommended. I knew they wanted me to get better, but no one had considered what that might entail. Everyone, including me, expected me to move to the mountains, get my ski adventure in, and then go to graduate school and move forward with a career.

"Really?" my mother asked when I said I thought the doctor was right. "Maybe you should just rest a few more weeks and see how you're doing."

"I can hardly get out of bed. I don't know how I'm going to be well enough to ski." It broke my heart to admit that out loud.

"Okay..." I knew my mother was shaking her hands, the way she always does when she is worried or shocked. She doesn't like surprises. "We've got a lot going on here," she said. My mother and stepfather were going through a tough time. He was dealing with his own medical issue of laryngitis resulting from spasmodic dysphonia. My half-sister Elizabeth was fifteen, an age that speaks for itself in terms of drama and chaos. My mother had been so compassionate on the phone since I'd gotten back to Colorado, listening to all my complaints, but the possibility of me coming to live under her roof for an indeterminate amount of time was a tougher pill to swallow. I knew she wanted to help me, but between chairing the English department at my old high school and the tumult at home, she already had a lot to handle. I clutched my stomach as we spoke, a pit of guilt gnawing at my gut.

My father and Janet offered for me to stay with them, promising to find me a good doctor in New York. I had a room at their house and they'd always made me feel welcome, but I had never been sick there, at least not for longer than a day or two. I wasn't sure what that might be like. Things were busy in their home, too. My father traveled often for work, and my half-sister Alaina was a junior in high school.

It was a privilege to have family who could help me out; many patients don't. Still, I paced around my apartment in Boulder, trying to decide where I should go, whose feelings might be hurt if I didn't choose their house, on which family I would be less of a burden. Had I already been married, or established with a career that offered disability, I would have had a support system other than my parents, but at my age and point in life, I was on my own.

My long-distance friends all wanted to help. Sharon offered for me to stay with her and her fiancé in New York. My college friend Elise invited me to her place in Washington, D.C. I was so touched by their support, but the doctor had warned that it could take a year, even two, to get over EBV. How long could I live on a friend's couch?

After a few days to get used to the idea, my mother called. "We're your family. When you're sick, your family takes care of you. So that's what we're going to do. You're going to come here, we'll get you to a doctor, we'll get you well and back on your way." She can be even more stubborn than I, so I knew better than to argue. All I could say, over and over, was, "I'm sorry. I'm sorry

I went to camp. I'm sorry I'm not better. I'm sorry you have to deal with this."

The roots of my constant apologizing had been planted years before, when my mother married my stepfather, who took us away from our sunny home with the johnny jump-ups to a house that was run by remnants of his own abusive past. To diffuse explosions, I learned to be good as gold, or to apologize quickly when I wasn't. Going back to that house would mean returning to that same environment. But my mom had always taken care of me when I was sick. And I wanted my mom.

After many phone calls to both families to sort out logistics, we decided to ship my dented Jeep cross-country. I would fly from Denver to New York. My father would pick me up at the airport, I'd spend a few days at their house, and then he'd drive me to my mom's. In the meanwhile, my mom was going to get the name of a doctor in the Hartford area. I only had a few days to explain the situation to my landlord and friends, pack, and sell my furniture.

Within hours of posting ads, people were knocking on my door, fighting like vultures over my belongings. By the next morning I was left with three barstool cushions, an entertainment center, and my bed. The living room seemed big and empty. I could see the outline of the couch because the carpet around it had faded from the sun, but there was no longer anything to sit on to look at the mountains. I felt as empty as the apartment.

My shoulders slumped as I stepped into the kitchen to make instant oatmeal. I looked around the barren space, wondering where I should sit to eat. Dejectedly, I picked up one of the discarded stool covers and placed it on the carpet in the center of the living room. I flipped on the TV and plopped down on the cushion, breakfast in hand. Morning cartoons sang from the television, reminding me of old nursery rhymes. Suddenly I was laughing hysterically as I realized that I was Little Miss Muffet, sitting on her tuffet, eating her curds and whey. I chanted the rhyme and giggled so hard I couldn't even swallow my oatmeal. I put the bowl down and shifted side to side on my sit bones, cackling uncontrollably.

"You're losing it, Jen Crystal," I said aloud, and the bubbling emotion turned into heaving sobs. I tucked my knees to my chest and wrapped my arms around them, hot tears dripping from my cheeks to my chin to my kneecaps. I cried until there was nothing left. Then I stretched out on my back, nestled the stool cover under my head, and drifted into a feverish sleep.

Heather came a few days later to pack up the rest of my belongings in big tubs that she put in the Jeep, along with boxes of clothes and my ski gear.

"What should I do about my bike?" I asked.

"It's not like you're going to be riding it anytime soon," Heather replied. "Why don't I store it in my garage?"

I nodded enthusiastically. I liked the idea of leaving part of my active self as collateral for my return.

On my last morning in Colorado, I forced myself to go for a walk. I felt that I should see my neighborhood and breathe in the fresh Rocky Mountain air one last time. If "can't" wasn't in my vocabulary, "should" was one of my top words, urging me to do things I wasn't physically capable of.

My walk only lasted one block. Every joint in my body hurt. The pulling sensation was stronger than ever, yanking my muscles and bones toward the ground. I didn't yet know the term post exertional malaise, which affects many people with chronic illness, especially those with Chronic Fatigue Syndrome/Myalgic Encephalitis. Research on long-haul COVID-19 would later prove to society what many chronic illness patients already knew: that forcing yourself to exercise when not feeling physically well enough only makes you feel worse.[i] At the time, I saw pushing through as admirable, even when it literally caused me to sink to my knees on a patch of grass at the edge of a nearby park.

I tried to look around and appreciate the blue sky above me, the sun cresting the foothills. I dropped my hands to the ground, feeling the early morning dew on my fingers. Grasping clumps of blades, I put my head down on the wet grass. The coldness was soothing against my fevered cheek. Curling into a fetal position, I started to cry again. "Please," I whimpered into the earth, "please let me get well. Please let me have made the right decision to go to Connecticut. Please let me get my life back soon."

---

i   https://pubmed.ncbi.nlm.nih.gov/36911963/

I slept through the entire flight to New York. When we landed, I trudged slowly through the bustling airport, wanting to shield my eyes and ears against the bright lights and crackling announcements. When at last I pushed through the doors to baggage claim, I saw my father's familiar trench coat, salt-and-pepper hair, and wire-rimmed glasses. He was holding a "Welcome Home" balloon. I waved and gave a wan smile but couldn't make my leaden feet move any faster.

My dad enveloped me in a hug. "I was wondering if I had the right carousel. Everyone else from your flight got here a while ago."

"I don't move very fast these days."

"Come, *Tatala*." My dad smiled as he used this Yiddish term of endearment. "Let's get you into the car." He hauled my bags off the carousel and took my arm, guiding me slowly out of the airport and through the parking lot.

I closed my eyes as soon as we got in the car. Resting my head against the passenger window, all I could think was, *I want to go home*.

CHAPTER 5

I got a referral to a primary care physician in Hartford. He flipped through my chart as he walked into the exam room where my mother and I sat waiting. "I see you had mono?" he asked, stroking his gray beard.

"I still have it." I told him what the doctor in Colorado had said, that the mono had slipped into chronic Epstein-Barr virus. I explained I wanted to get his opinion on that diagnosis and see if there was something else going on.

"It seems strange that someone your age wouldn't be able to fight off mono," the doctor said as he washed his hands. "It's very rare that cases actually turn into EBV."

I said that I'd gone to camp that summer and had probably pushed my body too hard.

"Even so," he replied, "you should be over mono by now."

He began a complete physical exam. His large hands felt cold and rough against my skin as he checked my glands and lymph nodes. "These all are fine." As he pressed on my stomach, listened to my lungs, and looked in my ears, I explained that my fatigue had gotten worse since camp. I told him that during my two years in Colorado, I'd experienced strange symptoms like hives, shaky hands, and hair loss, which my doctor there couldn't explain. I tried to detail the horror of my persistent nightmares, the pain of my aches, the burning in my feet. This doctor didn't say anything until he stepped back and looked at my face. "I see your eyes are two different shapes," he said. "Your right eye is wider than the left."

The left eye droop had developed after eye surgery to correct weak muscles when I was a senior in college. The ophthalmologist had said it was an effect of the operation. I thought the fact that this doctor noticed the droop meant he was thorough. However, his observation was merely topical. If he had looked deeper than my surface symptoms, considered a reason for facial droop beyond surgery, or tried to connect my current presentations to the unexplained ailments I'd experienced over the years, maybe he could have found what was really going on. Like so many patients in our fifteen-minute-exam-and-diagnosis medical system—especially young women, whose complaints historically were written off as hysteria and now are often seen as stress[i]—my full narrative wasn't being considered.

The doctor said he'd re-do the mono test and EBV titers, for good measure, and run labs for "all the major things," like lupus and cancer.

Out of the corner of my eye, I saw my mother gulp hard. "I have non-Hodgkins lymphoma," she said quietly. "It's in remission. Do you think she could have that?" I hadn't realized that my mom was connecting my medical situation to her own history, or considered how hard and scary this was for her, too.

The doctor shook his head. "No, I don't think it's anything like that. Don't worry," he assured us. "I'll get to the bottom of this."

A few days later his receptionist called with my blood results. "You have mono," she announced, as if she were giving me the answer I'd long been waiting for.

"I know."

"You know?"

"Yes. I've had mono since June. The doctor was looking to see if something else was going on. He was also supposed to check my Epstein-Barr titers."

"Your what?"

"Epstein-Barr titers. If they're high, it means I have an active

---

i   https://www.nytimes.com/2013/03/17/opinion/sunday/women-and-the-treat-ment-of-pain.html

infection." It made me nervous that I was the one explaining this to someone who worked in the doctor's office.

"Well, you definitely have active mono."

I sighed. "Yes, I know. Did the blood work say anything else? May I speak directly with the doctor?"

"The doctor isn't in," the receptionist said curtly. "All he said was to tell you that you have mono. So, make sure you rest."

I couldn't believe I was having almost the exact phone conversation I'd had back in June. With that nurse, I'd pleaded to have my life continue forward as planned despite the diagnosis of mono. Four months later, my life seemed to be moving backwards.

Returning to my childhood home as an adult was out of order of the way things should be. Being under my parent's roof made me naturally slip into my old role as a child, but I wasn't a kid anymore. I was an adult who had already lived independently, and I adamantly wanted that life back, especially now that I was once again under my stepfather's wrath. I tried to play my old parts, helping my mother around the kitchen and my sister with her homework, but besides the fact that I was too sick to be of much use, they didn't necessarily want or need me in those roles anymore. When I asked how her math test went, Elizabeth told me she didn't need two mothers. The curtain had closed on the life I'd been a part of in that house, and a new family dynamic had been established in my absence when I moved out many years before.

Elizabeth was only eight years old when I left for college. Though I'd been home for visits, I hadn't lived there for any extended period since then, and it took some time for us to figure out what it meant to live in adjoining rooms at fifteen and twenty-five. Elizabeth liked to talk on the phone late into the night, just as I had when I was her age. Her bedroom wall backed up to mine. When we were younger, Elizabeth and I used to knock on that wall to send each other secret codes. Now, I knocked to ask if she could lower her voice, a request that usually elicited banging and yelling. No teenager wants to be silenced by anyone, especially an older sibling who isn't otherwise supposed to be around.

I needed TLC, and while my mother did her best to give it to me, the fact that I needed it at all made everyone in the house anxious. I'd come to Connecticut to get answers. A continued prescription of "rest" was hardly the fix-all we'd hoped for. How long would it take for me to get better?

Day after day I awoke feeling exactly the same: like I had a terrible case of the flu. No amount of sleep helped, and the smallest effort, whether it was checking the mail or going to the pharmacy, sent me back to bed for hours. I was sick and tired of looking at the same four walls of my bedroom, sick and tired of being sick and tired.

My aunt Nancy, my mom's twin sister, bought me a picture of the Rocky Mountains to put next to my bed. Every morning I saw that photo as soon as I woke up and told myself that I would someday get back there. Then I'd sit up and see my college diploma hanging on the far wall across from my bed. At first it made me proud, but as the weeks wore on, I was ashamed to look at that marker of my past achievement. My father had worked his whole life to send me to a good school, and what did I have to show for it?

As I lay in bed, I often heard my stepfather yelling in the kitchen, telling my mother that I was lazy, that I obviously didn't want to work or be a responsible adult. His accusations reminded me of the time when I was thirteen and my lips swelled up like a duck's bill from an allergic reaction to pumpkin. Not even looking at my face, he had said, "Well, are you just pushing your lips out? Are you faking it?"

I wasn't faking it at thirteen and I wasn't faking it at twenty-five, but I didn't have the energy to fight back. All I could do was rest, but with the sense that my presence in the house was only adding to my family's stress, I couldn't get the respite I needed.

My mother suggested I call the doctor's office again. "See if you can get him on the phone. Tell him you aren't getting any better. Maybe he'll have some new ideas."

But he said exactly what the doctor in Colorado had. "Mono can take a really long time, especially when it's slipped into active EBV."

My shoulders sank. "When I came to see you, you thought it was unlikely that someone my age would have EBV. Are you sure there isn't anything else going on?"

"All your other tests came back negative." The doctor deferred to "cookbook medicine" which, as described by Drs. Leana Wen and Joshua Kosowsky in *When Doctors Don't Listen*, is a reliance on heavy algorithms and tests that assume patients should fit a certain "recipe."[ii] When they don't, some 25 million Americans are left with undiagnosed diseases.[iii] "It is rare," the doctor continued, but it seems you just have a very bad case. I'm afraid I can't tell you much else to do but rest."

I was sick of hearing that word. "What about vitamins? Or dietary changes?"

"Well, have you cut back on your water consumption?" The doctor had been alarmed when, during the appointment, I'd told him about my excessive thirst; I could easily drink 16-20 glasses of water a day.

"I can't," I said. "I'm really that thirsty. I feel dehydrated and headachy if I drink any less."

"You're not supposed to drink that much. Maybe try some hard candies when your mouth feels dry."

I rolled my eyes. "What about food?"

"Eat things low to the ground."

"Low to the ground?"

"You know, like turkeys and chickens and plants. Those are healthier."

It was hard not to burst out laughing.

"One more thing," he said before we hung up. "I think you should see someone to talk about your feelings."

Anger gurgled inside me. In college, health center nurses had grown tired of my frequent visits for my on-and-off flu, eventually suggesting, "Maybe you should see someone in Counseling about all of this." At such an impressionable age, I wondered if they were right; maybe my illness was psychosomatic. As a result, I worked harder than ever to sweep symptoms under the carpet, to pretend I was fine when I wasn't, to get right back to a tumultuous schedule, the only pace of living I'd ever known.

Recurrent flu-like symptoms and the uncertainty and angst they caused may very well have impacted my mental health during

---

ii   Wen, Leana, M.D. and Kosowsky, Joshua, M.D. *When Doctors Don't Listen: How to Avoid Misdiagnoses and Unneccessary* Tests. New York, Thomas Dunne Books, St. Martin's Griffin, 2012 (3).
iii   https://commonfund.nih.gov/diseases

my college years. It probably would have helped to speak with someone. But there was far greater stigma around mental health then, especially as an effect of physical illness rather than the cause of it. At that time, I saw the suggestion of counseling as code for, "It's all in your head."

But this doctor's voice softened when he said, "It can be hard to be sick for so long, especially at your age, and you might want to talk to someone about that."

He referred me to a psychiatrist whose office was as old and stuffy as she. Her only acknowledgement of my physical illness was to ask if I had a living will. Then she switched gears, inquiring if I was on the substitute teacher list at any of the local schools, in a tone that told me what the answer was supposed to be. I wanted to shout, "I wish I could be on a sub list, but I barely had the energy to drag myself here!" But I could only mutter, "I feel so tired, there's no way I could substitute teach."

"Well, you should get yourself on a list," the doctor said matter-of-factly, as if I'd mumbled nothing at all, as if the pale, sleepy-eyed young woman in front of her was a robust, rosy-cheeked, insolent child who just needed to be scolded into behaving. "It'll give you energy. You'll get up and moving."

She also recommended I buy a workbook for people with social anxiety. Being tossed out of my life made me vulnerable and insecure, and I was sensitive to everything anyone said to me, even these insensitive doctors. I began to wonder if I was just anxious. Maybe my stepfather's accusations were true. Maybe I couldn't handle being a responsible adult. I was too exhausted to think clearly, so I turned to the suggested reading for answers. The exercises were for people who feared going out in public or had trouble associating with their peers. I shook my head as I skimmed through the book, thinking of how easily I'd always made friends, how much I loved to go out and do things in all the places I'd ever lived. The book wasn't for me, and I gathered the strength to tell the psychiatrist that when I next saw her.

She slammed her hand on the arm of her chair. "These exercises are very helpful to all of my patients." I wondered, then, in what group she and the referring physician had categorized me. How many other young adults with mysterious ailments were thrown into this same category? And what did that say for those actually suffering from mental illnesses, whose very real diagnoses were used as a catch-all for anyone who didn't fit a standard recipe?

The psychiatrist played with a thick locket that hung over her droopy bosom. I wondered who was locked inside. I reached up and fingered my camp necklace, tracing the outline of the water-skier at its center. I vowed to get her back into the forefront of my life, no matter how long it took. Not just for me, but for all those in the same position. Our voices deserved to be heard.

CHAPTER 6

Months of monotony passed. I felt as if I were stuck in the flats between two ski slopes, struggling to move myself along. I migrated between houses, sometimes staying with my dad and Janet for a few weeks and also spending time at my aunt Nancy and uncle Steve's. Tension between my mother and stepfather had risen to fever pitch. Nancy and Steve offered me harbor in a beautiful guest bedroom adorned with my favorite colors: purple and yellow. When I slept there, I imagined what my future bedroom, my future house, could look like. I just couldn't yet imagine feeling well enough to live there.

I saw infectious disease doctors, internists, and rheumatologists. One read aloud about mono from a dusty medical textbook. Some said chronic EBV didn't exist. Others told me to exercise. I tried in vain to explain how active I used to be, how badly I wanted to live that high-functioning lifestyle again, but that I felt too sick to do so. I sensed most of the practitioners either didn't believe me or thought if I simply worked harder on a mind-over-matter mentality, I would be fine.

I used to think doctors had all the answers. A doctor was supposed to be a wise elder figure like my pediatrician, Dr. Werner. In his sixties at the time, with a white moustache and a reassuring voice, Dr. Werner brought calm into the examination room. He always acted like it was so good to see me, like he knew everything about me, and from a child's perspective, that made him trustworthy.

At twenty-five, I was too old for a pediatrician, but I didn't know where else to turn. How could I trust the doctors who came into the room trailing impatience, never looking up from their charts, calling me by my last name? In cookbook medicine, doctors often interrupt patients within the first thirty seconds of a clinical encounter.[i] They start with the chief complaint and then follow a diagnostic and treatment plan from there, without taking the full patient history into account.[ii] These doctors all promised they would get to the bottom of my symptoms, but then ran the same blood tests and said there was no answer besides mono. The disconnect was vast between what I said and what the doctors heard.

Email became my lifeline, a way to stay connected with friends and tell them exactly how I was feeling. As I typed, a dull ache ran down my forearms, into my palms, and up each finger, as if little Epstein-Barrs were scurrying through me, searching for an escape. I wished they'd pop right out of my fingers and run away, but short of that happening, I put the invaders to work writing about the havoc they were wreaking on my entire being.

My friend Patrick, a.k.a. "Paddy," started an online support group for me with Elise and some of our other college friends. One day he wrote, "Jen, the matchmaker of hope and effort, what can we say about you? It's been a hard road since last spring—leaving Colorado, the hurt of a loved one, season-upon-season mono, and a diagnosis of Epstein-Barr. You have shown me how to remain sweet, without bitterness, toward life. 'Well, I slept for four days straight, but I felt good yesterday, and drove myself to the post office this morning!' Who else but you, Jen? We are all standing beside you. We are holding you close as news comes from doctors and hold you in loving arms as you lie down to rest, and smile and sing with you as you greet the day."

One day I ran into a childhood friend's mother at the post office. She was surprised to see me in town, knowing I had been in Colorado. As we waited in line together, I explained why I was in Connecticut.

---

i   https://jamanetwork.com/journals/jama/article-abstract/2635621

ii   Wen, Leana, M.D. and Kosowsky, Joshua, M.D. *When Doctors Don't Listen: How to Avoid Misdiagnoses and Unneccessary Tests*. New York, Thomas Dunne Books, St. Martin's Griffin, 2012 (4)

"But you don't look sick," she said. It was a comment I heard often from well-meaning people. I tried to make myself presentable when I went out in public, at least changing from sweatpants to jeans and sometimes even applying makeup. Putting myself together made me feel more human, but it also made it harder for others to understand what was going on inside my body. When I'd torn my ACL, I'd had props to prove that the tear had not occurred in my head. The visible nature of the injury made it real. Acceptable. Admirable, even. At the time, I'd thought it was the worst medical adversity I'd ever deal with, but actually it was the best, because it wasn't questioned. Years later, I'd get that same appropriate response when I got COVID-19, because everyone understood what the illness entailed, and everyone's life was on hold because of it. With EBV, as with other invisible illnesses, there isn't that solidarity.

In line at the post office, I told my friend's mother that mono had slipped into chronic EBV.

"Well, you're at the post office," she quipped. "Can't you just send it away?"

I thought of that conversation many times as the seasons slipped by. Winter came, and with it the explicit knowledge that I wasn't going to make it back to Colorado anytime soon. I thought about a ski day during my final year teaching in Colorado. The school where I'd taught offered experiential learning trips, and another teacher and I had taken a group of students to Crested Butte for an avalanche awareness course. Crested Butte has the steepest ski run in the United States. The students called it Crusty Butt. I called it impossible.

"C'mon Ms. Crystal, you can do it!" the students had called up from the bottom of the biggest mogul field I'd ever seen. Below me were not just bumps, but mounds of snow that were as high as my hips. The students and our guide had bounced right through the field and were huddled together at the bottom, waiting.

I stood at the top trying to see which moguls I could bounce off to create a line. But all I could see were the deep crevasses in which I was sure to fall. There was no place to bail out of the mogul field if it got too hard. We were essentially skiing on rock face that happened to be covered in moguls. On either side of it were sheer drop-offs that would lead to certain death.

I attempted a series of false starts. I would push off, then turn a sharp right to stop myself. With each semi-turn, I was creeping closer and closer to the edge. When I'd ski instructed on weekends in high school, I'd always told kids that in the worst-case scenario, they could take their skis off and walk down. There I was, in front of my own students, seeing no alternative. Until that moment my skis had always seemed an extension of my body. I could control them on virtually any slope, often without thinking. Standing at the top of that mogul field, the sport became far more cerebral than it had ever been. The anxiety in my head took over the comfort in my feet, which felt, for the first time since I was a child, wobbly and disconnected from the boards to which they were attached.

Pressing my poles against my bindings, I released my boots from my skis. I lifted the boards up over my right shoulder, held both poles in my left hand to steady myself, and skidded down the field by the bottoms of my boots. The whole scene went completely against my nature. I remembered the banner that had been waiting at the bottom of the hill when my college classmates and I came down for our celebratory graduation run: "Some were born to walk. Others were born to ski." I may have come down that graduation run in a sled, but I was not born to walk.

Lying in bed in Connecticut, I wondered, *What if I can never ski again?* I allowed my mind to slip to a scarier question. *If I'm no longer a skier, who am I?*

Hope came in early spring. An acquaintance of my father's recommended a naturopathic physician in their area. Since I wasn't getting anywhere with conventional medicine, I was more than willing to give the holistic method a shot.

Dr. Taylor's office sent an intake form for me to fill out before my first appointment. I wrote out my medical history starting from the first low blood sugar reaction at camp in 1997. It took four single-spaced pages to record everything that had happened in the subsequent six years. I was tired of repeating the story to doctors who didn't seem to have, or didn't want to give, the time to listen. Penning my full history validated my persistent illness in writing. As I sat in Dr. Taylor's waiting room a few days later, I clutched the papers to my chest as a shield against the hopelessness, fear, and frustration I'd taken away from so many other appointments.

Dr. Taylor read every word I wrote. I could hear the clock on his office wall ticking as I sat in the chair next to his desk, watching him furl his thick eyebrows. He pushed back in his rolling leather chair, playing with his red tie. "I see you've been on antibiotics a number of times over the years."

"Yes. I've had so many ear infections and sinus infections, and a couple cases of bronchitis."

Dr. Taylor frowned. "Antibiotics can destroy the good bacteria in your intestinal tract. Did you take probiotics while you were on them?"

I'd never heard of probiotics.

"Show me what you mean by a pasty white tongue," Dr. Taylor instructed.

I stuck out my tongue, instinctively saying, "Ahh."

He looked in my mouth. "That looks like a candida infection." He explained that without probiotics to counter them, antibiotics can cause intestinal yeast overgrowth, also known as candida, which disrupts the integrity of the gut and can spread to a systemic infection that often manifests in bad breath or a white tongue.

"But I haven't been on antibiotics in a while."

"Candida can also be a result of diet. Do you eat a lot of sugar or yeasty foods?"

Sheepishly, I informed the doctor that I was a chocoholic, and that I loved bread products.

He nodded. "I'll run a candida test to be sure, but I'm going to suggest that you go gluten and sugar free right away."

"You mean, I can't eat chocolate?" My eyes widened. "I don't know if I can do that."

"A systemic candida infection weakens your immune system," Dr. Taylor said. "It may be the reason you get acute infections so often, and it's probably exacerbating your fatigue."

I sat back. If giving up chocolate meant getting back my energy, I could try it. At least for a little while.

Dr. Taylor then proposed other reasons I might not be getting better, despite months of rest. He didn't discount EBV, but also wanted to consider underlying conditions such as thyroid or adrenal dysfunction or autoimmune disorders. I felt he was getting closer to the root of the problem than any other doctor had.

"It's like a light has been shining on only one place, so that's where everyone has been looking," Dr. Taylor said. "I want to look around in the dark now and see what else is there."

That night at dinner I was excited to tell my dad, Janet, and Alaina about Dr. Taylor, but by the time we gathered around the round glass table for tacos, I couldn't remember half the things he'd said. Relaying the doctor's words to my family was like playing a game of telephone. By the second recount when I called my mother later that night, the information was even fuzzier.

I wished someone would offer to go to doctor's appointments with me, to write down notes and help ask questions. Because I was an adult, I think my family was afraid to step on my toes. By the same rationale, I was scared to ask for help. Our little dance left us not really knowing what the other was feeling or experiencing, all of us just waiting for the day when I would be back to my usual self and on my way again.

The candida test indeed came back positive. I ate a last supper of ravioli and chocolate fudge brownie ice cream, and then went cold turkey off gluten and sugar. At first, I craved my favorite foods, but after a few weeks, I grew accustomed to the new diet. I started thinking about what foods would nourish my body, like fruits and vegetables, lean proteins, and complex carbohydrates. My blood sugar crashed far less frequently, and even though I was still sick, I felt nutritionally well.

Dr. Taylor's tests also showed that my adrenals were shot, which he felt explained my prolonged fatigue. He diagnosed me with Chronic Fatigue Immuno Deficiency Syndrome, or CFIDS, now more commonly known as Myalgic Encephalomyelitis/Chronic Fatigue Syndrome (ME/CFS). Marked by intense fatigue, post-exertional malaise, unrefreshing sleep, concentration problems, and pain, ME/CFS affects up to 3.3 million Americans.[iii] Dr. Taylor put me on a regimen of Chinese herbal pills, homeopathic supplements, and acupuncture.

---

iii   https://www.cdc.gov/me-cfs/index.html

I wanted so badly for the treatments to work. In part, they did. Acupuncture helped me relax. I imagined the needles pinpointing all the little Epstein-Barrs, sending them scurrying in fright. I visualized health and good energy flowing through me. But despite my best intentions, I couldn't will the treatments to fully eradicate my fatigue.

My father went out and bought me every book he could find on CFIDS. I read them all, but my family didn't read any, which only deepened the divide between what I needed them to understand, and what they saw and wanted. I felt terrible that I wasn't getting better fast enough, an anxiety that certainly didn't help the balance Dr. Taylor wanted my body to achieve. He prescribed a low-dose anti-depressant, but it didn't do much to alleviate my deepening despair.

My college friend Elise provided greater calm than any medication could have. After college, she'd been sidelined from her adult life for two years with a traumatic brain injury, the result of a biking accident that almost killed her. Doctors were shocked by her survival but told her she would never fully recover. At the time, only half of her brain was functioning properly; she struggled with fine and gross motor skills and intense fatigue. She understood my situation because she had lived it. And she'd defied doctors' expectations and she'd come out the other side.

"I know it doesn't seem like you're doing anything when you're just waiting to get better," she told me. "But your body is working really hard to repair itself. It needs this time to heal."

I wrote Elise's words down and taped them to my bedroom wall, not only as a reminder to myself but also in hopes that my family would read them. Elise had moved forward in spite of a bleak prognosis. Somewhere in me remained the little flicker of hope that I could, too.

Soon after my twenty-sixth birthday in May, I received notice of an opportunity to take summer courses at the Bread Loaf School of English in Vermont. Affiliated with my alma mater, the Bread Loaf campus was near the mountain where I'd been pulled down in a sled for my mid-year college graduation. I looked at the glossy brochure for the six-week summer program.

The idea of being back in an environment I loved, engaging

with people my own age on my favorite topics of literature and writing, seemed like the perfect tonic. My family agreed. This idea fit within the productive, successful narrative my life was supposed to follow. Had I not gotten sick, I would have been just finishing up my ski adventure and either looking to start graduate school or a new job. I felt like my year of being sick was "up," even though I wasn't better.

I was offered a scholarship, so the chance would provide us all a break without financial burden. Perhaps, we all secretly wished, I would get my health back while I was there. Maybe I would even make contacts that would help me find a job in a post-sickness world.

Dr. Taylor was not as supportive of the idea. "You really need to rest," he cautioned. "If you went away somewhere, it should be to a retreat where you could just relax, and someone would bring you your supplements and pills."

"This will almost be like that. If I'm too tired to go to class one day, I'll skip it. And I promise to take all my pills."

My pleading the previous summer had been to get to camp so the forward motion of my life would not be halted. Now I'd come to a near standstill, and I needed a way to jump-start my existence again. When Dr. Taylor told me to think of my energy in terms of savings, not credit card spending, I assured him that going to Bread Loaf would be a real investment in both my health and my future.

"Well," he said warily. "Good luck."

CHAPTER 7

I pushed open the creaky back door to the main building of the Bread Loaf campus. As I stepped onto the gravely path, I stumbled over a wooden ledge in the door frame. A member of the administrative staff was coming in and caught me before my books and I tumbled to the ground.

"You must be tired today," she said with a wink. I'm sure she thought I'd been out partying the night before, like most students my age.

"Well, I have Chronic Fatigue Syndrome."

"Oh!" The woman gasped, tucking her hair behind her ear. "I'm sorry. I didn't realize. I…"

"It's okay," I said quickly, and hurried away.

Recalling that conversation years later makes me cringe with second-hand embarrassment for my twenty-six-year-old self. I'm mortified by my self-absorption, by my need to tell everyone who crossed my path about my situation. I'm humiliated by how much I stuck out at Bread Loaf as the "different" one. I was one of the only students with a single room, having brought a doctor's note saying I needed too much rest to have a roommate. The dining hall made me special meals, using supplies I'd brought. On the first day of class, my professor asked everyone to describe the community in which they served, since most of the other students were teachers during the year. I stammered when it was my turn, not sure if I should describe my former school in Colorado, or my current community which consisted of me, my family, and a sickbed. I went with the latter because it had become my chief identity.

I'm embarrassed that I was known as the sick girl. And I also have empathy for my younger self, seeing just how mired I was in my world of illness.

The class focused on ways to engage young people in purposeful writing. The lessons made me realize that even if I were bedridden, I could still write. I considered writing some essays about my experience to help others going through it, but I was too close to the situation to take on that task effectively. All that came out was one list:

I Wish 7/2/04
I wish I could be sitting outside writing with everyone else
I wish my body wasn't achy and feverish
I wish it weren't an issue to walk up a flight of stairs
I wish I could stay up all night writing a paper, just because I could
I wish people could see on the outside how my body feels on the inside
I wish I could take an energy pill that would make my fatigue go away
I wish I hadn't gone to camp last summer
I wish I could go for a run
I wish I could water-ski
I wish my body was well enough for my mind and heart to be light

One day my mom called to say she'd run into a high school classmate of mine. "Do you remember during your senior year when her mother had Lyme disease?" my mom asked breathlessly.

"Kind of...?" The classmate and I had played field hockey together. I vaguely remembered her telling me that her mother had been bitten by a tick while vacationing in Old Lyme, Connecticut.

"I remember the whole family was on a strange diet." I paused. "Actually, I think it's the diet I'm on now."

"Exactly. She was bedridden for a year, just like you."

"Really? I don't remember that."

"Yes. She said she was so achy and tired, and the kids all had to pitch in."

My pulse quickened. "So, what are you saying? I should get tested for Lyme disease?"

"Can't hurt, right?"

Even though I'd worked in the woods at camp and grown up in Connecticut, home to the town for which the disease was named, I hardly knew anything about Lyme.

When Alaina was eight months old, a tick had left a bullseye rash behind her right ear. I remember her pediatrician saying how lucky she was that she'd been diagnosed and treated immediately, because the disease could become very serious.

Janet had brought Lyme up once in the last year because she'd met someone whose son was suffering from it. I remembered her saying that doctors had finally discovered this boy had Lyme when they tested his spinal fluid, because it could be hard to diagnose. I hadn't given much thought to the story at the time. But now I wondered if I had ever been tested for it. Lyme was a bacterial infection, and that meant it could be treated. With newfound hope, I slipped flip-flops on my feet, raced out of the main building and across the street to the infirmary. Anyone who saw me must have thought it was an emergency. Anyone who knew me must have wondered where I suddenly got the energy to run.

I blew into the little yellow infirmary cottage. I recognized the woman there as one of the many health center nurses who had seen me during my college days. She motioned me into a wooden chair next to her desk below a big window that faced the road. "What can I do for you?"

"I think I might have Lyme disease!" The pronouncement came out with such excitement that the nurse eyed me curiously.

"Were you bitten by a tick? Did you find a bullseye rash?" She was as soft-spoken as I remembered from college.

"No." I sat forward. "But my mother just talked to a friend whose mother had Lyme disease and she said my symptoms are just like hers. I'm wondering if maybe I've had Lyme all along?" My words came out in a jumbled rush as I tried to explain why I would want to have an illness. "There's no treatment for the condition I've been diagnosed with, Chronic Fatigue Immuno Defiency Syndrome, but there's treatment for Lyme."

"Oh…" The nurse looked up at me with a sudden recognition that made my cheeks burn. "I remember you from your undergrad days."

Immediately my stomach tensed. Was she going to suggest I see someone in Counseling again? I quickly said, "So my symptoms sound similar to my friend's mother's. Could I have Lyme?"

No one had asked this question when I first took sick during sophomore year of college. Since being diagnosed with mono, I'd been so intent on convincing people that my EBV was not laziness that I'd stopped pressing for doctors to look any deeper, to consider if something additional might be going on.

The nurse agreed to run a test. Neither of us had any idea that there were different types of tests with varying levels of accuracy, or that many Lyme patients never find a tick bite or bullseye rash, leaving them in the same position as me: sick, confused, and maligned for years on end. If we had, we might have pushed beyond the basic test she ran, which came back negative. Instead, I took the result at face value, once again feeling dejected and stuck.

By the end of the summer program, I had created an online portfolio, the 2004 version of a personal website. It showcased my past writing, my teaching philosophy, and my interest in the intersection of the two. Online I sounded like a well-qualified writer and teacher, but in person I was a disintegrating body who didn't have the strength to put those ideas into practice. I wondered how I would ever lead a purposeful life. If I could barely manage one class, would I ever be able to do the Ph.D. program I'd once dreamed of? A year had been hard enough on my family and me, but what if my illness went on infinitely? What if I never got better?

My professor suggested I become a Writer-in-Residence in an inner-city school. She was willing to connect me with teachers in New York and even help me get a grant to write a book about my experience in their classrooms. The opportunity sounded incredible, but I was starting to come to terms with my limitations. If I could only spend a couple hours in a class that was right on campus, how would I possibly last a full day at school in New York? I would have to commute an hour by train from my dad and Janet's. All of that was way beyond my realm of ability, no matter how badly I wanted to take the job. I was finally learning to say "no" when I wanted to say "yes."

My dad, Janet and Alaina came to pick me up from Bread Loaf in August, using the trip as part of Alaina's college tour. It was strange to think that my kid half-sister was old enough to be looking at schools. At nine and ten years my junior, she and Elizabeth had always seemed so much younger than me, but I sensed that gap closing. They were almost the age I was when I was last truly healthy.

We drove away from Bread Loaf, down into town. I knew it would be impossible for me to walk the span of the campus, so my family dropped me outside the student center on the main quad. I pointed them in the direction of the Admissions Office, where they could catch a guided tour of my former life. It seemed absurd that this campus I'd once raced across to get to class and run past to get to a three-mile jogging trail was now too big for me to handle, no matter how slowly I walked.

I looked up at the gray stone buildings that had been mine to live and study in for four years. My gaze lifted to the top of the hill, atop which sat my sophomore year dorm. My face fell. That was the year I was first sick, wrestling severe flu-like symptoms and frequent low blood sugar reactions following the first one the summer before at camp. When I really thought about it, that was when my illness journey began.

I didn't want to revisit my sophomore dorm, but I did want to see the chapel next to it, the spire of which had served as a beacon on many cold undergraduate nights. The marble chapel stood tall and proud as ever, the colorful flags above its front door swaying in the breeze. I took a few steps toward the path that led straight uphill and quickly felt achiness in my legs.

This is ridiculous, Jen Crystal. It's just a few hundred feet. You can walk up that hill. I inched along until I reached the base of the path. Then my body protested, asking me to sit down. *You should be able to do this,* my mind replied. There was that dangerous word "should" again, tugging at the rift between mind and body, between desire and capability. *You walked this hill several times a day in college and thought nothing of it!* I looked down at my feet, wondering how I had ever gotten into this position. If someone had told me back when I was a student government representative and a campus reporter and a double major and a skier and a runner that someday I would be agonizing over walking the path toward the chapel, I would have laughed. Now I wanted to cry.

Slowly and deliberately, I put one foot in front of the other. I remembered my favorite English Professor John Elder reading aloud from his Introduction to Thoreau's "Walking": "Left foot/right foot, the walker moves through the landscape. Right brain/left brain, sensation and reflection flicker into the complex wholeness of human response."[i] I whispered the words aloud as I moved forward, concentrating on the sidewalk under my shoes that grounded each step. Every few feet, I stopped to rest. I refused to look behind me, because I was afraid I'd allow myself to believe I'd gone far enough. I didn't want to accept a mediocre view. *Left brain/right brain*, I tried to bring balance to a mind and body that were completely out of sync.

Halfway up the hill, I stopped and opened my side-slung bag to get my water bottle. I took several gulps, wishing I had the water backpack I used to wear skiing. I remembered how in sync everything had felt when I skied in Colorado, how naturally I'd been able to create momentum. Would I ever get that back?

I looked up, noticing the psalm etched in marble above the columns on the front of the chapel: "The Strength of the Hills is His Also." I'd always wondered what the phrase meant and why it was on our non-denominational chapel. The college is surrounded by the Adirondacks and the Green Mountains, so I'd vaguely interpreted the quote to mean that the beauty of those hills was not just the school's, not just the students', but that of a higher power. That interpretation humbled me and rang true when I considered the spiritual home I'd found among those mountains while I was in college. Now, the psalm seemed to be a message of faith.

When I finally reached the top, I turned around and immediately broke into a wide grin. The view was more beautiful than I remembered. Before me was a clear picture of the campus I loved. From the top of the hill, I could see the leaves of the magnolia

---

i   Elder, John. Introduction. *Nature Walking*. By Thoreau, Henry David. Boston: Beacon Press, 1992 (xiii). Nature Walking originally published 1918.

trees falling softly on the grass, and in the distance, I could make out the peaks of the Green Mountains. "Home," I said softly, then again loudly, because I didn't care if anyone heard me. I spread my arms wide. "HOME."

I sat down on the cool chapel steps to rest and survey my old campus. I smiled wistfully, recalling the innocence and excitement of my freshman year, before I got sick. I shifted on the steps, thinking about the later college years. My senior thesis came to mind, a creative essay about the last year of my maternal grandmother's life. She and my grandfather had visited me freshman year, walking the campus with greater ease than I had on my trek up to the chapel.

Grandma had died the summer after my sophomore year. Folding my hands around my knees, I realized that freshman year stood out not only as a time before I'd been hit with physical illness, but also as a time before I was touched by loss. It was the time I most associated with Peter.

Peter Westra had been larger than life in my freshman eyes. Six-foot-three with jet black hair that hung in wisps across his forehead and a bright red ski parka that I could see coming from a hundred feet away, he lit up every room he entered. I remember walking into parties with him and the whole place would erupt in a cheer of, "Westra!"

He first walked into my freshman room after an intramural hockey game. A mutual friend Peter knew from home had put us in contact the previous summer. Peter and I had emailed throughout the fall—the yesteryear version of online dating— as I got ready for my mid-year matriculation. When I first saw him in person, I knew my life was about to change forever. He walked into my room with a huge grin and a mischievous sparkle in his soft eyes the color of a hazy summer day. We talked for hours, which turned into late nights on the phone, a movie in his dorm, a game of croquet in two feet of snow at 3:00 in the morning, midnight sledding runs...

I refocused my gaze on the path below the chapel and giggled, recalling a winter night when Peter had come up behind me, picked me up, and thrown me down in the snow. I remembered a similar time when he stole my winter hat and I ran after him down the hill, both of us laughing as we chased each other until we again landed in each other's arms in the snow. Sitting on the chapel steps, I could still feel that red ski parka scratch against my cheek. I could still feel the weight of his chest and the heat of his breath. I could still feel his strong arms dipping and twirling me at a Valentine's Day dance.

I stretched my pale legs in front of me and placed my hands flat on the chapel steps, letting the cool marble bring me to the present. I sighed, wishing I could go back.

I had no way of knowing the role Peter would come to play in helping me move forward.

CHAPTER 8

"We have your salad," my dad said to me one morning when I groggily walked into the kitchen for breakfast. I had been living at my dad and Janet's for most of the fall following Bread Loaf. My mom and stepfather's relationship had hit a final breaking point. He'd walked out for good, and my mom was going through the proceedings of a divorce. Since my dad and Janet's house was closer to Dr. Taylor's office, it made the most sense for me to shift my home base there.

"What salad?" I asked, opening the refrigerator to get some orange juice.

"The one you ordered last night while Janet and I were out for pizza."

I stared at my dad, utterly confused, until slowly, like a drunken memory, the night started to come back to me. Since finishing Bread Loaf, I'd been wrestling insomnia. Dr. Taylor's naturopathic suggestions of melatonin and special herbs did nothing to quiet my brain, so he eventually gave me a non-narcotic prescription sleeping aid. It did the trick. It also, apparently, made me silly enough before I fell asleep that I decided to "drunk dial" the pizza place, order my favorite salad, and ask the waiter to deliver it to my parents' table so they could bring it home for me.

We got some good laughs out of my antics, which gave levity to the underlying tensions of, when would I get better? How long would this go on for? Would I ever get out on my own again?

Though I knew my family meant well, I got tired of being asked how I was feeling every day, because EBV, like other chronic illnesses, doesn't improve on a steady continuum like strep throat or the flu. I might feel some improvement one day and then completely crash the next, a spiraling process that left us all exasperated. Pre-COVID-19, my family and society at large didn't understand an indefinite pause, especially since it wasn't collective. As with COVID-19, after a while, we all got tired of the situation and just wanted life to resume.

I did my best to be as productive as possible with my limited energy and unreliable schedule. I didn't feel comfortable just staying home and watching *The Price is Right*. I felt pressure to be productive, to prove my worth, as any young person suddenly sidelined from life would. Though I hadn't been able to take my Bread Loaf professor up on the offer to be a Writer-in-Residence in New York, I was able to serve in that role remotely for a local classroom. High school English students of a teacher I'd met at Bread Loaf posted their creative writing pieces to a class blog, and I commented on them. The exchange proved fruitful for us all. The students were more willing to share personal pieces with someone they'd never met, and I was able to give my best editing skills without having to show my sick face. When I had to nap for three hours between essays, no one knew.

My camp friends Kendra and Rachel both lived nearby and took me out for lunch every few weeks. They reassured me that the real Jen Crystal was still in there and it was just going to take a little longer for her to come back. They kept the faith I'd felt that summer when climbing up the hill to the chapel, but as the months grew longer and we headed into another winter, I started to lose my own.

One January morning, I decided to blow dry my hair, something I rarely did. Holding my arms up over my head to shake the hairdryer was painful and tiring. Perhaps I had a spurt of energy that morning. Perhaps I was going to lunch with the girls and wanted my hair to look normal, not pulled back in the usual messy bun that made my head look like an egg. Maybe I was cold.

Whatever the reason, the signs that day were large and clear: big red rashes on both elbows, which I never would have seen in the mirror had I not lifted my arms to dry my hair. They were circular red marks that looked suspiciously like the classic bullseye rash of Lyme disease.

"Maybe I was leaning on my elbows too hard, and left a mark," I suggested to Dr. Taylor at an appointment a few days later. So many doctors had written my symptoms off that I had learned to do the same.

But Dr. Taylor shook his head. "I think you should be tested for Lyme disease."

"I was tested for Lyme over the summer. It came back negative."

Dr. Taylor explained that standard Lyme disease tests are notoriously inaccurate because they only look for antibodies against Lyme, not for the bacteria itself. He recommended I see a Lyme specialist, who could do more sensitive testing and make a clinical diagnosis. "Look, I've been treating you for two years," Dr. Taylor said. "If it were only EBV, you'd be getting better. I've started to suspect an underlying infection, maybe something that was going on before you had mono, maybe since your sophomore year of college when all your symptoms began." Dr. Taylor knew I had something outside his scope of care, and when he couldn't solve it, he acted in the best interest of his patient and sent me to someone who could.

Southern Connecticut is teeming with ticks, the vectors of Lyme, and therefore is home to some Lyme specialists. I was referred to Dr. Raxlen, a world-renowned psychiatrist who had backed his way into this specialty when more and more patients written off as psychosomatic landed in his office. It turned out many of them were actually suffering from late-stage neurological Lyme disease, which, once it crosses into the central nervous system, can have psychological manifestations. By the time I saw him, Dr. Raxlen had been treating the neuropsychiatric and neuro-cognitive complications of tick-borne diseases for almost fifteen years.

All patients did their initial intake with the doctor's Physician's Assistant, Natalie, just a few years older than me. She greeted me in the waiting room with a solid handshake, then led me to an exam room and had me sit in a chair next to her desk. "I just want to talk to you first, before I examine you."

I liked her immediately. She and I both knew that she was the medical practitioner and I was the patient, but she sensed that in order for that relationship to work, she was going to have to earn my trust. Unlike so many doctors I'd seen before her, except for Dr. Taylor, Natalie wanted to take the time to get to know me and my medical history. She had already read my whole chart.

"It seems like you've been through quite a lot," she said. "It's clear to me, just from reading these notes, that something long-term and systemic is going on in your body. My job today is to hear the whole story, from you, and then to evaluate if you might have tick-borne disease. Does that sound okay to you?"

That sounded more than okay. That sounded unlike anything any other mainstream doctor had ever said to me.

I described to Natalie the on-and-off flu that plagued me in college; the high susceptibility to bronchitis, ear infections, and sinus infections; the systemic hives; the joint and muscle pain; the achiness that seemed to pull my body down onto my bed; the smashing migraines; the burning extremities; the insomnia; the hallucinogenic nightmares; the crushing fatigue; the night sweats; the constant low-grade fever; the mono that had slipped into chronic Epstein-Barr virus and never gone away. Natalie occasionally asked a question, but the narrative was mine, so mostly she just listened and recorded.

When I finished, Natalie read through her notes. "Your story sounds similar to that of many patients I see," she said. "Most people with late-stage Lyme and other tick-borne diseases missed the original rash, or never had one at all, and never got diagnosed properly." She explained that without treatment, the Lyme bacterium, called a spirochete, self-replicates and spirals into every system of the body, twisting its way into bones, muscles, and cells, sometimes crossing into the central nervous system.

She asked if I'd ever seen a bullseye rash before the ones I noticed on my elbows. I started to shake my head, but then remembered the blotchy red dots I'd found on my right forearm back in 1997. I remembered showing it to the camp nurse, remembered how quickly she'd passed it off as nothing. Natalie said that a Lyme rash, called erythema migrans or EM, doesn't always look like a bullseye; it can also be red and blotchy. "EM rash can appear months or years after the initial tick bite, and can present in various places on the body," she explained. "Your blotchy rash was the same summer you developed hypoglycemia?"

"Yes."

"Which came first, the rash or the low blood sugar reactions?"

"The rash was towards the beginning of the summer. The first low-blood sugar reaction was mid-summer, probably in July."

"Did you ever think to relate the two?"

I shook my head. "Neither did the camp nurse, or anyone since then, though."

Natalie nodded. "It's okay. This is why we're here today, to piece everything together. In addition to Lyme, I also want to test you for co-infections. Ticks don't just transmit Lyme disease, unfortunately. A single tick bite can deliver several different pathogens that can cause infections such as babesiosis, ehrlichiosis, and Rocky Mountain Spotted Fever."

That last was the only one I'd ever heard of, since it was fairly common in Colorado. The others did not even sound like English. Natalie reassured me that my lack of awareness about co-infections was common, accounting for thousands of mis-or-undiagnosed cases. People being treated for Lyme disease who have not been tested for co-infections may only be fighting half the battle, Natalie cautioned. "For example, babesiosis is a parasitic infection that usurps the oxygen in the red blood cells. It needs to be treated with anti-malarial medication." She said the parasite can cause low blood sugar, migraines, and the feeling of 'hitting a wall' during exertion.

I sat forward in my chair, rapt, even though we were talking about serious medical conditions. "Sometimes," I stammered, "when I try to exercise or even move too much, I feel like my arms and legs are having a panic attack."

Natalie laughed good-naturedly. "What exactly do you mean by that?"

"My arms and legs feel shaky and jumpy, like they're missing something. Like they need blood, or water, or…"

"…Or oxygen?"

"Yes! Almost like I'm not getting air to my limbs. And when that happens, I always get a migraine." I pointed to my left eyelid. "It starts here, and then then moves up over my head—"

"I read in your chart that you've had eye surgeries to correct weak muscles," Natalie noted. "Spirochetes love to congregate in scar tissue, so it's possible you have more scar tissue over that left eye."

I remembered that it had taken my knee much longer than expected to heal from ACL reconstruction. Maybe spirochetes had been living in the scar tissue there, too.

Everything was starting to come together. No other doctor had offered an explanation that so closely matched what I was experiencing, that accounted for all the weird symptoms that had accumulated over the years. Each and every symptom I described fit one or more tick-borne disease. Even the hives pointed to systemic inflammation. And the sleep disturbances and other neurological issues "might be a sign that Lyme has crossed the blood-brain barrier," Natalie said, "but let's not jump to any conclusions until we run some tests." She explained that the blood-brain barrier is supposed to protect the brain from infection, but that spirochetes are smart and persistent and can sometimes break through, making Lyme much more difficult to treat.

"Let's do some basic cognitive tests," Natalie suggested. We started with easy memory exercises. Natalie said three numbers or words and asked me to repeat them back to her. I did these without a problem. But then Natalie gave me an idiom, "A rolling stone gathers no moss," and asked me to tell her what it meant. I stared at her. I blinked several times, realizing that I was taking too long to answer. I knew I had heard the phrase before, but I could not come up with its meaning. "Is it a song lyric?"

"Let's try another. How about, 'A chain is only as strong as its weakest link.'" This one I knew. I started to feel a little better, though I couldn't shake the fact that I'd drawn such a blank on the first one.

Finally, Natalie had me change into a gown and hop up on the exam table. The white paper crinkled beneath me, a noise that had become part of the soundtrack of my life. These exams were so routine that I could anticipate which step was coming next. I'd hold my arm out for the blood pressure cuff, then offer my wrist for a pulse check. I breathed deeply before the cold stethoscope touched my chest, swallowed hard for thyroid checks before the doctor's fingers massaged my throat, stuck out my tongue and said "ahhh" with much greater willingness than I had as a child.

Reflex tests were not always part of this routine. They were something I associated more with childhood exams, remembering how my pediatrician Dr. Werner used to tease me for responding so well to knee taps that he was afraid I would kick him. I was surprised, then, to see how slowly my reflexes responded to Natalie's taps. My legs and arms gave delayed, tiny reactions, an external representation of how tired and slow I felt on the inside.

"Maybe it's because I had my ACL repaired a few years ago," I suggested to Natalie.

"Have you had a problem with your reflexes since then?"

"I don't think so, though maybe they haven't been tested for a while." I did have a problem of explaining away what was happening to my body, a problem of trying to find a way to say—or to agree—that everything really was fine.

Natalie pursed her lips and scribbled something. Then she told me she was going to check certain pressure points on my chest and back that are strong indicators of Lyme. Using her thumbs and the tips of her fingers, she pressed on the points one at a time. I yelped in surprise when she tapped the first one.

"I'm barely touching you," Natalie said. "That's just how sensitive these points are."

"It feels like you're hitting a bruise."

The whole exam took close to two hours. Natalie took her time reviewing her notes. I swung my legs like an impatient child, noticing how dry and pale they were. I wondered when I'd last cut my toenails.

Finally, Natalie spoke. "Based on everything I've seen and heard today, I suspect that you have been battling tick-borne illness since summer 1997, when you found that rash on your arm and developed hypoglycemia. My guess is that your immune system was slowly weakening over time as the infections spread, and that when you got mono in 2003, your system became so overtaxed that the underlying infections came out in full force."

"So, I have Lyme disease?" I said excitedly, as if I was saying, "So, I won the lottery?"

"That is my clinical suspicion," Natalie said. "Your tests will come back in a couple weeks. I'd be highly surprised if they came back negative. So surprised, in fact, that I'm going to start you on treatment today." She wrote a prescription for a month's worth of antibiotics. "If they don't work, we can always stop."

After such a thorough exam, I trusted Natalie's expertise. "How long do you think it will take for me to get better?"

"Well, you've been sick for a very long time. Tick-borne illnesses that are caught right away and treated as soon as a rash or symptoms are discovered can often be cleared up in three weeks. But yours have been festering in your body for eight years."

I felt the hair stand up on the back of my neck. "So, if I'd been treated back in the summer of 1997, I would have been fine?" I looked at Natalie's legal pad, the pages and pages of notes documenting everything I'd been through since then, all the result of a bug smaller than a poppy seed.

"Well, we can't say for sure, because your tests might have come back negative then." Since it can take the body a while to build up antibodies, many people get false negative test results early in Lyme infection. And we now know that of those who are diagnosed and treated early, 10-20% still go on to have persistent symptoms.[i] I also might not have been evaluated for co-infections even if someone had considered Lyme disease back in 1997. "Still," Natalie said, "if you had been accurately diagnosed and treated at the time, we probably wouldn't be here today dealing with all of this."

We were both quiet as I attempted to digest the fact that a three-week course of medication eight years earlier might have changed the course of my life.

"Even though you've been sick for a long time, you're already ahead of the game in terms of treatment," Natalie broke the silence. She said she would have recommended the gluten-free, sugar-free diet I'd been following under Dr. Taylor. She explained that both sugar and gluten can exacerbate inflammation, and since antibiotics can cause intestinal yeast overgrowth, it was good that I was already on a diet that countered that risk. Natalie handed me the prescription. "This infection could clear up in three months. Let's start with this, wait for your labs to come back, and go from there."

---

i   https://www.lyme.health.harvard.edu

I was ecstatic. Three months was nothing compared to the two years I'd already lost to being sick. I might even be able to start working soon! Or go to graduate school! My mind spun with the possibility of living again—something I hadn't considered in my perpetual ghost-like state of survival—and I wanted to run outside and shout from the rooftops, "Hey world! Guess what? I have Lyme disease!"

If only I'd known what that really meant.

PART II

CHAPTER 9

The sound of the shower woke me from a jumbled dream. For a moment, I didn't know where I was. Then I heard Alaina clattering her makeup in the bathroom and remembered I was in my room at my dad and Janet's house, where the head of the bed backed up to the wall between my bedroom and the bathroom Alaina and I shared. Alaina was getting ready for school. It was time for me to get ready to face another day.

I lay still. I wondered how a person could be alive when her body was lifeless. I'd wondered this nearly every day since starting antibiotics six weeks earlier. I'd expected the medicine to slowly clear up my symptoms, the way they work on a sinus infection or bronchitis. But within a week of beginning treatment, I started feeling worse than ever.

"This is great news," Natalie said. "It means the medicine is working. Stay the course."

Natalie explained that I was having a Jarisch-Herxheimer reaction, when bacteria die off at a faster rate than the body can eliminate them, making the patient feel worse before better. The reaction confirmed what Natalie said my blood work had overwhelmingly shown: I had a very clear case of Lyme disease. I also tested positive for the co-infections babesiosis and ehrlichiosis. The latter could be helped by antibiotics, but the former required a liquid anti-malarial medicine that looked and tasted like bright gold paint. At night, I sweated out the dead parasites, often waking two or three times to change my soaked pajamas.

The dead spirochetes left my body in a different way. Hearing Alaina finish up in the bathroom, I mustered the strength to raise my head off the pillow, then slowly pushed up on my elbows. A deep ache pulsed from my neck to my appendages as I creaked upright, dropping my feet to the carpeted floor. I suddenly felt what had become a familiar urge and knew I had about three seconds to get to the bathroom.

Wobbling with dizziness, I walked across my room as quickly as I could, holding the doorframe for support as I stepped into the hallway and turned left into the bathroom. I barely got my nightgown lifted and underwear down before my bowels exploded. The release came with the rush of diarrhea but the consistency of foam noodles snaking out of me in long tubes. The toilet filled so quickly that I had to flush before continuing to go. I gagged when I caught a glimpse of my stool, which I can only describe as toxic waste.

After washing my hands, I limped back to bed. Sinking into the pillows, I wished I could retreat into a dream world, despite the fact that sleep was not always a good escape from reality. Even with sleep medication, my hallucinogenic nightmares persisted. Sometimes, though, I was graced with my old healthy body in my dreams and got to ski, travel, or spend time at camp. The dreams were vividly detailed and incredibly accurate. I might walk across Paris and see all the shops, people, street corners, and sidewalk cracks I'd known when I studied abroad; I might explore a cave in an Eastern European city I'd never visited in real life, and then look that city up in the morning to find that my "vision" of it had been correct; I might ski so hard that I'd wake with sore legs, my thumbs still curled around my dream poles.

Camp was a recurring theme. One night I dreamed I was walking across the camp's beach toward the water-skiing cove. My dream body was not tired as I reached the end of the beach and turned onto the path in the woods that led to the dock. As I rounded the corner, I saw Kendra coming back from parking the boat. Her tanned arms swung purposely by her sides. They were the kind of arms that could wrap a homesick camper in a bear hug, pick up a canoe by the mid-ship thwart and throw it over her shoulder like a laundry bag, or burst out of the water in a beautiful butterfly stroke.

"Yaya," Kendra said, our standard greeting we'd borrowed from the eponymous movie about four childhood girlfriends who were as mischievous and full of life as we were in our camp counselor days. Kendra lifted her sunglasses.

"Yaya." I lifted my glasses in turn.

Kendra opened her right palm to reveal a crumpled granola bar wrapper. "THIS is nonsense."

I giggled sheepishly. "Well, if I drive the boat for three hours in a row, my blood sugar gets low. You don't want me to pass out at the wheel, do you?"

"So you put the wrapper in the steering wheel?"

The steering wheel had a wooden center console that unscrewed, leaving what seemed to me the perfect place to store things, both in real life and, apparently, in my dreams. "Well, I didn't want it to fly into the water," my dream self said.

"No, instead it flew out and hit me as I was driving!" Kendra was trying to sound like she was chiding me, but she was grinning. "Yaya," she said again, shaking her head as she pulled her sunglasses back down. We high-fived as we passed each other and continued in opposite directions, she treading in my footprints back to the beach and I tracing her steps to the dock.

These dreams made me feel connected to my old self, the person Kendra and Rachel believed was still bottled inside my sick body. Dreams of camp reminded me of the role that place had played in developing my zest for life. Above my bed hung a frame of the camp emblem, similar to the outline of my ten-year necklace. I'd received the emblem at sixteen when I became a Counselor-in-Training. Underneath it was a quote from the camp's founder, describing the ideal camp girl. "…She is full of the love of doing things, and she sees the humorous side of life. We admire serious girls, but we adore girls brimming over with the joy of being alive."[i]

Camp was the place that had given me life, but it was also a place I associated with death. On July 8, 2001, the summer after I graduated from college, I stopped in the counselor hut on my way to teach rowing and saw a big message scrawled on the white board by the phone: "Jen: call Alix ASAP."

Alix was a college friend who was working a high-powered investment banking job. She never had time to make phone calls, especially during the day. My stomach lurched as I pulled my cell

---

i   Charlotte V. Gulick (Hiiteni)

phone out from where I stored it in a cubby. There were three missed calls from Alix. She'd left one voicemail simply asking me to phone her. I mentally flipped through our mutual college friends, wondering whose parent might have died.

I was going to be late for rowing, but I dialed Alix. She answered on the first ring. Her voice sounded soft, but it was a Monday morning and she was at work, so I figured she had to whisper.

"Is everything okay?" I rubbed my left hand across the edge of the bright orange beach towel folded around my waist.

Alix did not pause. She simply said, "No, no it's not."

I lifted my hand to the wooden window ledge that overlooked the camp's playground, bracing myself. But I never could have been prepared for the words that came out of Alix's mouth. "Peter Westra was killed on Saturday night."

I can still feel the rough edges of the window ledge as my hand slipped from it—in fact I can smell the wood itself—and I can still feel the saggy green cushion of the chair into which I sank. I remember looking up through the window and thinking, *But it's sunny out.*

The rest of the conversation is a blur. Alix continued speaking softly, calmly, as my body trembled. I don't recall exactly what she said, but I do remember it took me awhile to ask, "Wait, what happened? Was it a car accident?"

For the first time, Alix paused. "No...no, it wasn't an accident."

I must have gulped. I think I was already crying. I remember clutching my stomach and rocking back and forth as I asked, "So what happened?"

I don't know how Alix managed to maintain such a controlled voice as she said, "He was beaten to death outside of a night club."

I stood up. "What???" Blood drained from my head, and I had to sit right back down. At this point a few other counselors had trickled into the hut and were looking at me curiously. I ignored them.

"They were at Brad's bachelor party..." Sweet, fair-haired Brad, Peter's sophomore year roommate who had once walked in on us watching a movie and had simply stuck out his hand to introduce himself.

"They were in Atlantic City, out of their element. For some reason Peter was ejected from the club and tried to go back in to get his credit card. He was met by bouncers who beat him repeatedly and kicked him in the head until he died."

"What? Why would he have been ejected?"

"We don't know yet." Later an investigation would conclude that Peter had been groping the dancers. When a bouncer had talked to him, likely about that, Peter had apparently put his hand on the bouncer's shoulder. I could picture him doing that, saying, "Hey man, I'm sorry." Whatever transpired—whether Peter even actually touched the dancers, we'll never know for sure, only that all the guys were drunk—instead of simply calling the police, the bouncer put Peter in a headlock and dragged him down the stairs. He then placed Peter on the hood of a car and roughed him up. When Peter tried to get back in the bar, six men emerged: the original bouncer, the owner, the manager, and three other bouncers. They all kicked Peter to death, with the original bouncer kicking him in the head football-style.

In the counselor's hut, I sobbed and shook. The only thing I remember Alix saying is, "There's some solace in the fact that he was unconscious, and probably didn't feel any pain." I took no solace in this as my own pain seared through my gut. Years later, perhaps I could. But in that moment there was no solace for anyone, not for me, not for Peter, not for his parents...*oh God, his parents*. I pictured them in their home in Minnesota. I'd visited Peter and some other friends one summer but had never met his parents. I thought of the kind, salt-of-the-earth people of that Midwestern state and wondered how they would ever make sense of such news.

To me it made no sense. Nothing did. Not the saggy green cushion, not the beach towel around my waist, not the concerned counselors rubbing my back, offering to make me tea. Eventually two of them took me under my arms, the way an injured athlete is carried off the field, and walked me up to the infirmary as giggling campers ran past. I never made it to rowing.

I didn't make it to the funeral, either. It was impossible to get that time away from camp. I also wasn't sure if it was even my place to go. Four years had passed since the semester I'd spent time with Peter. For the rest of college, our time together had fizzled to quiet lunches and awkward hellos, and we'd only been in touch sporadically after graduation. Each of us had moved forward from that innocent semester to different lives. At the time of his death, Peter was working as an investment banker in London. He was distant from my life, but still sometimes present in my thoughts. In the quietest, safest place within me, a place no one else could see, I sometimes still wondered—hoped—there might be a chance for us to reconnect in the future. As I lay on an infirmary bed reeling from Peter's death, that quiet, secret place whispered, "And now that chance is gone."

I gave myself the rest of that day to grieve. I went for a drive, which was probably not the safest plan, and blared songs I associated with Peter. I cried. I screamed. And then that night I went back to the cot in my bunk, forcing a saccharine smile for my campers and pretending that everything was fine. The next day I resumed camp activities. I made it through each day by remaining viscerally in the present of that summer. But at night, in rare moments by myself, I was haunted by the ghost of memories past.

I thought about the past a lot as I lay sick in Connecticut, nearly four years after Peter's death. I looked at pictures of happier, livelier times for tangible reminders that I was once a healthy, spirited person. In addition to emailing friends about my physical illness and the emotions surrounding it, I started writing to them about fun memories we'd shared. I typed out brief anecdotes from my time studying in Paris, like the time I waited all day for a plumber because my French toilet had a broken "motor," or the time my friends Chris and Pete cooked up a sizzling science experiment of bright green chicken. I laughed aloud in bed, a sound I hadn't heard in a long time.

CHAPTER 10

After six weeks of Lyme treatment, I finally met Dr. Raxlen. For the first and last time for a while, my dad, Janet, and my mom all came with me to the appointment. Everyone wanted to meet the Great Oz.

The office was adjacent to an exam room and set up like a study, with cases of medical textbooks and a desk piled high with papers. As we took seats, I glanced at the row of framed diplomas and awards on the far wall. Dr. Raxlen sat in a big leather chair.

"Well kiddo, it seems you're pretty sick." He patted my huge file with one hand and waved my blood work with the other. Ordinarily if someone called me "kiddo" it would feel condescending, but the way Dr. Raxlen said it, it made me feel like he was in my corner. He spoke not just to me, but to my parents, scanning his eyes between us the way a good teacher does in the classroom. "Your daughter's tests indicate both IgM and IgG antibodies for Lyme disease. IgM antibodies usually indicate a newer infection and IgG antibodies indicate an older one. What that means is she was probably infected in 1997, as Natalie surmised." I was pleased to hear that either Natalie had briefed Dr. Raxlen, or he had read her notes. "But Jen may have been re-infected at a later point. Or the infection is just so active right now that the tests are giving us a short-term read." From the get-go, Dr. Raxlen admitted that so much of Lyme diagnosis and treatment is educated guesswork.

He turned to me. "You were back at the summer camp after 1997, right?"

"Yes. I was there from 2000 to 2003."

"And you've been living in Connecticut, one of the most endemic areas for Lyme in the country. For all we know, you got another tick bite here." Dr. Raxlen paused to let the irony of this statement settle around the room.

I had a feeling, though, that if I'd gotten a second tick bite, it was probably at camp. Besides the fact that I never wore bug spray and walked through the woods every day, there was also the issue of how I spent my nights off. We counselors told the campers that we went bowling; amongst ourselves, we called it "bowling for boys." In quintessential summer camp romance fashion, we spent our nights off with counselors at a nearby boys' camp. The girls would pile into my Jeep, Kendra sitting shotgun, Rachel scrunched in with various other counselors across the backseat. It wasn't uncommon for a few people to sit in the way back with the six-packs of hard lemonade and empty beer bottles clunking around.

The boys had a bonfire at the edge of their woods, away from the bunks. We traded stories while someone played guitar. Every so often one of our counselors and one of theirs would disappear into the woods together to "collect firewood." Before I moved to Colorado and met Jim, I had a camp boyfriend. We met in 2001, just before Peter died, and for two summers we got naked together either in the woods or on a deserted field. We thought to use condoms but not to do tick checks. We didn't think of much beyond looking at the stars as strums of music and wisps of pot smoke drifted up in the distance.

Janet broke my reverie. "The Lyme test Jen had done last summer was negative."

Dr. Raxlen explained that the test I'd had at Bread Loaf was only a first-tier ELISA test. The CDC recommends a two-step test for Lyme disease, starting with an ELISA that looks for antibodies against the bacteria. If that test is positive, they'll move to the second test, which at the time was always a Western blot test (and now is sometimes a second ELISA test). Because it can take a while for antibodies to build up in the blood, the first ELISA test can often give a false negative read. Many patients who do have

Lyme are simply told their results are negative and are never given the second test. That second Western Blot test looks for reactivity against different proteins, called bands, found on Lyme bacteria. By CDC standards—which were originally created for surveillance, not diagnostic purposes—two of three IgM bands or five of ten IgG bands must be positive for a test to be considered overall positive. A person who tests positive for three or four IgG bands will be told they don't have Lyme disease, even though they do show antibodies against Lyme bacteria.

"Tests can be a helpful part of the diagnostic process, but they certainly aren't the sole way to know whether a patient has Lyme," Dr. Raxlen said. "In your case, we have the blood work to back up the clinical diagnosis. Yours is a CDC-positive test. There's no question at all that you've been harboring tick-borne diseases for a long time."

I looked at my parents. They sat quietly, staring straight ahead. I shifted in my seat. My right leg suddenly jolted like it'd been given a reflex tap.

"Do you get those twitches often?" Dr. Raxlen raised his chin in the direction of my leg.

"Mostly when I'm overtired, which is often," I tried to joke. "Or sometimes when I'm trying to fall asleep, or when I'm watching TV."

Dr. Raxlen stroked the facial hair on his chin. "Those are typical signs of an inflamed neurological system." He turned to my parents. "The Lyme bacteria, spirochetes, are smart little buggers. They spiral away from antibiotics, burrowing deep into cells, bones and, often in long-term cases like your daughter's, the central nervous system." He turned back to me. "The achiness in your forearms—would you say that's muscular?"

I shook my head. "It feels deeper than that."

"Damn bugs have probably gone into your bones."

"It has gotten a little better since starting treatment, though." After a few weeks of intense pain, the achiness throughout my body was dissipating.

"The aches are always the first to go. Sometimes you will still feel pain deep in your bones, though, because the antibiotics have chased a few spirochetes in there."

Janet sat forward and pushed her glasses up with the knuckle of her right index finger, her signature habit when she's thinking something through. "So let me understand this," she said slowly. "We've got Jen on these really strong antibiotics, and the medicine is just pushing the infection further into her body?"

"I understand why that might seem counter-productive," Dr. Raxlen said. "But this is a really serious multi-system infection that your daughter's fighting, and the only way to kill spirochetes is with heavy-duty antibiotics. Without them, Jen's symptoms would only get worse, and the infection would continue to spread. With them, we can at least start to fight some battles in this war."

Janet nodded.

"However," Dr. Raxlen continued, "many of the spirochetes *are* dying, which we know because of the improvement of Jen's achiness and because of her...how did she phrase it?" He flipped back through his notes and smiled slightly. "Toxic waste."

"But the medicine's not getting all of them," my father stated.

"Unfortunately, no," Dr. Raxlen replied. "So we will keep fighting them, keep chasing them, until we get this girl back on her skis."

I sat back and uncrossed my legs, comforted by the fact that Dr. Raxlen understood what part of my identity was missing here. I looked at the doctor. "So, if my neurological system is inflamed, does that mean the Lyme has crossed the blood-brain barrier?"

"What's the blood-brain barrier?" all three of my parents asked in unison.

"The blood-brain barrier is supposed to protect the brain from bacterial infections," Dr. Raxlen told them. "It's like a security guard for the central nervous system. With long-term, serious infections like we're dealing with here, that security can be compromised. Once the spirochetes enter the central nervous system, the disease becomes much harder to fight."

Dr. Raxlen leaned down and shuffled through some papers on the floor next to his desk. From a large manila envelope, he pulled out what looked like X-rays. "Your MRI results look pretty good." He held up the transparent pictures of my brain. I'd had the MRI taken not long after I saw Natalie. "I don't see any lesions, which is a good sign."

My parents and I relaxed a little, though we could hear a "but" coming.

"But the twitching, as well as the burning sensations Jen's experiencing in her extremities, and, of course, her sleep disturbances, are all neurological manifestations of this disease. I'd say there are some bugs in that brain, but we'll focus on quieting them down." Dr. Raxlen added, "As neurological symptoms go, it could be a lot worse, and Jen is actually pretty lucky. Eight years is a long time to go undiagnosed, but there are patients who go fifteen, twenty years without a diagnosis. When tick-borne diseases are unchecked for that long, they can cause paralysis, schizophrenia, and even death."

A hush fell over the room. Dr. Raxlen was used to saying these words, but for my family and me, they spelled out the direness of the situation. For me they also, ironically, led to some relief, because they made me consider what might have happened if I had stayed in Colorado and the spirochetes and parasites had continued to run rampant.

"So, what are the next steps?" my father asked, always looking for a plan of action.

"Well, in a case this severe that isn't clearing up with oral antibiotics, I might recommend we go the intravenous route. That will help us start attacking some of these co-infections better, too."

I glanced nervously at my parents. An IV? Would I have to be hospitalized?

"I know this sounds daunting," Dr. Raxlen said, "but it's the fastest and most effective way to get at these infections. It will also take the pressure off Jen's gut." He turned to me. "Even though you've been taking probiotics and an anti-fungal to avoid a *C. diff* infection, and sticking to the gluten-free, sugar-free diet, your digestive system can really take a beating from long-term oral antibiotics."

In lieu of a central line directly in my heart, as many cancer patients use, I would get a peripherally inserted central catheter, or PICC line. The line would run up the inside of my arm and across my chest to pump the medicine to my heart. "You'll self-administer the antibiotics twice a day," Dr. Raxlen said.

My eyes widened. "To my heart? Is that safe? I'm not a nurse!"

"But there will be a nurse who teaches you how to do everything, who will come to your house once a week to check your line and change the dressing."

This news assuaged me only a bit.

"There is some risk with an IV," Dr. Raxlen warned. "The line can clot, but a nurse will always be on call to take care of that. The medicine I'm going to put you on can cause gallstones, but that's very rare."

The room was still as we all digested this information.

"You can take some time to think this over, and let me know how you want to proceed," the doctor said.

My mom asked, "If Jen did this, how long do you think it would take for her to get better?"

Janet piped in, "Yes, Natalie had initially hoped three months on the orals, and obviously that didn't work."

"Some patients do clear up in three months, and that's what Natalie was hoping for when she gave you that prognosis," Dr. Raxlen replied. "That was before we had the blood work and knew what kind of co-infections we were dealing with. Unfortunately, with tick-borne diseases, every case is different. There's no set treatment protocol. I can see a thousand patients with a thousand different manifestations. Treatments that work great on one patient might totally miss the mark with another."

Hearing the number "a thousand" reminded me just how many patients Dr. Raxlen had treated. I trusted that he knew what he was doing, or was at least going to give it his best shot.

"Let's do it," I said firmly. I looked at my parents for validation. They didn't seem to know what to do or say, but they weren't disagreeing with the decision, either. I think we all felt that if this more extreme treatment might help, we were willing to give it a try.

As we stood to exit, I repeated my mom's question. "So how long do you think it might take?"

"I don't want to put a timeframe on it, and have you get attached to that," Dr. Raxlen said. "Let's just try this for a couple months, see how you're doing, and then reassess." He opened the office door to usher us into the hallway. "I'll be honest. This is a pretty serious case. It's going to be a long road ahead."

CHAPTER 11

I sought a second opinion from another reputable Lyme specialist, who read my blood work and agreed with my diagnosis. He didn't use intravenous antibiotics in his practice, so his recommendation would be to treat me orally. Despite the potential risks, I wanted whatever medicine was going to help me the fastest, so I chose IV. A nurse put the line in at Dr. Raxlen's office, giving me instructions as he stuck a needle in the crook of my elbow. He slowly threaded a catheter from insertion point through the interior of my arm and across my chest cavity. I felt it slither under my collarbone. I grew sweaty as the line headed towards my heart. "Are you sure this is safe?"

"I've done this many times," the nurse assured me. "But just to make sure I placed it accurately, you're going to get a chest x-ray at the hospital."

The X-ray checked out, and I returned to the office for my first dose, watching with a mixture of fascination and fear as the nurse showed me how to extend the external tubing of the line down my left arm until I could secure the end of it in my palm; then twist its little blue cap off with my left thumb and forefinger while simultaneously unscrewing the cap of the bolus, or balloon-shaped ball of liquid antibiotics, with my right hand; then attach the ball to the open line. Within minutes, the medicine was pumping into my arm and heart, though I couldn't feel a thing.

Each morning, I hooked a bolus to my PICC line and let it drip for an hour while I sat at the kitchen table, left arm extended. When the ball deflated to a flat bag, I used my right hand to flush the line with syringes of saline and heparin to make sure it didn't clot.

The nurse had cautioned me not to get even a drop of water on the line, and to pump the medication slowly. "It takes an hour because you don't want to push liquid into your heart too quickly. Be sure to push the saline and heparin very slowly, too, or you'll really feel it." I learned this the hard way one night, when I became too confident in the process and pushed the heparin in impatiently. I felt a cool rush in my chest, and then heart palpitations and sudden dizziness that sent my head below my knees.

That episode scared me enough to endure the painstakingly slow process, which felt like the medical manifestation of watching paint dry. I was usually alone for the morning infusion, reading emails or the paper as I sat with my arm extended across the kitchen table. After infusing and flushing the line, I wrapped the external portion of the IV cord around my elbow and stuffed it into a mesh sleeve that fit over my bicep and forearm. At night my family, whichever one I happened to be staying with at the time, watched game shows with me to help pass the infusion time. I shouted the answers to *Wheel of Fortune* puzzles and *Who Wants to Be a Millionaire?* questions, wishing I could become a contestant and spin my way out of this mess.

One day a check for over $20,000 arrived in the mail. For a minute I thought I'd won the lottery, but then I realized it was insurance reimbursement for one month of intravenous antibiotic treatment. Flabbergasted, I mailed the check to Dr. Raxlen's accountant, who told me I was extremely lucky to live in a Lyme endemic state, so my insurance company categorized long-term antibiotic treatment as emergency medication and covered the expense in full. Patients in other states were fighting uphill battles against insurance companies that denied treatment. They hid behind CDC guidelines, which at that time stated that all cases of Lyme could be treated with three weeks of antibiotics. This was true for cases that were detected immediately, but three weeks of antibiotics hadn't touched an advanced case like mine. The CDC guidelines were based off recommendations by the Infectious Disease Society of America (IDSA), an organization stacked with doctors with significant conflicts of interest, including ties to insurance companies that profit from a denial of chronic Lyme disease.[i] Dr. Raxlen was a member of the International Lyme and Associated Diseases Society (ILADS), a group of Lyme-literate physicians whose guidelines recommend treating the patient for as long as needed, based on the doctor's discretion.

Despite my good fortune of living near an ILADS doctor and getting coverage for the most expensive portion of my treatment, I still had co-pays and out-of-pocket costs that gnawed a hole in my bank account and a pit in my stomach. The many nutritional supplements I took to boost my immune system weren't covered at all. My father was generous enough to help, and I was so grateful for his willingness and ability to come to my aid. Needing that help in the first place, though, made me very uncomfortable. As my friends got promotions and mortgages, I worried that I'd never be able to support myself again. I, like so many other people who have lost their independence for any reason, lacked agency.

I spent hours, and energy I didn't have, writing appeal letters to insurance when they refused, again, to pay for one of my oral medications or one of my doctor's appointments. I applied for Social Security disability benefits, a laborious process of confusing paperwork that ended with a big red "Rejected" stamp. The fatigue induced by these stressors only exacerbated my symptoms.

Every afternoon I laid down for a nap, but my brain rarely turned off. While my body was in park, desperate for rest, my brain was in overdrive, firing with songs and ideas and thoughts that swirled over each other like three movies playing at once. There was no question that the neurological symptoms of Lyme disease were getting worse. After a few months of IV antibiotics, I could no longer watch game shows, because I developed brain fog that felt like my head was full of cotton. The flashing images on TV were too bright and loud. I tried reading magazines but had trouble comprehending a simple story. I was getting migraines at least two or three times a week. I pictured the spiral-shaped spirochetes flaring in anger as the antibiotics chased them through my brain. I visualized the "Herx" as dead spirochetes clumping like piles of mud in my head until my body could eliminate them.

i   https://underourskin.com

"You're still making good progress," Dr. Raxlen told me at my spring appointment. All three of my parents had decided to come with me, something they hadn't done since my first appointment, because they were anxious about my worsening symptoms. "With a serious, multi-system inflammatory infection like this, it takes time, and unfortunately healing isn't a linear path," Dr. Raxlen told them.

My dad glanced at Janet. "These naps Jen takes every afternoon," Janet said. "Is she hurting herself by doing that? I heard a segment on the *Today* show that napping isn't good for you, because it can interfere with your ability to sleep at night. Maybe if Jen was up more during the day, she wouldn't have trouble sleeping." The question came from a lens of health, not of illness. I finally had understanding from my doctors, but my family still inhabited the un-paused world I once had. Not having experienced persistent illness themselves—even my mom's Lymphoma had been treated, thankfully—and not having yet lived through a pandemic where they were forced to reckon with a complex illness ravaging a population, they were having a hard time seeing life from my perspective.

Dr. Raxlen calmly told them, "Jen is lying down in the afternoon because she is just that sick. She needs the rest to get well. If she pushed through those times, I can guarantee you her night time sleep would get worse, because her body and brain would be that much more over-tired."

Janet pushed her glasses up and looked at my dad.

"And you feel the PICC line is the best choice for her," he stated.

"Yes. She's doing great on it. The ups and downs are to be expected, but she's certainly made a turn towards improvement."

"Any sense of how long…" my dad trailed off, waiting for Dr. Raxlen to fill in the blank.

"We can't really say, but she's doing well, and we'll know when the time is right. For now, she just needs to stay the course so she can continue getting well. If we pull the line out too soon, she could go backwards. I'm sure you don't want that to happen."

My parents didn't want that to happen, but they did want the forward progress to move faster. I did, too, but I was taking what I could get since I was the one sharing the body with the bugs that were slowing my healing, my progress, and my life.

I began seeing a therapist named Michele. After my negative experience with the stodgy psychiatrist who had brushed off my illness and told me I had a social anxiety disorder, I'd been hesitant to seek other mental health support. Between Paddy and Elise's email group, daily phone calls from Sharon, calls and cards from friends from all walks of my life, and visits from Kendra and Rachel, I wasn't sure I needed professional psychological help. But as time wore on, I was willing to give it another try.

Michele's office was the antithesis of the original psychiatrist's. A matronly woman with silver hair, pink cheeks, and shining eyes, Michele greeted me warmly and invited me into a cozy space. I finally saw the couches I'd always pictured in a therapist's office. Michele had a legal pad, but she set it to the side as she explained to me that the first appointment was just for us to get to know each other and see if we were a "match."

"There has to be a level of trust and comfort established between the patient and the therapist," she said. She looked directly at me as she spoke. "You need to make sure you're comfortable with me before we can dive into any of this stuff"—she motioned to the blank yellow paper—"and if you're not, that's absolutely fine. I can help you find someone who might be a better fit."

I liked Michele right away, just as I'd immediately liked Natalie. Michele had worked with Lyme patients before, and she had nothing but compassion for my situation. That isn't to say she coddled me. Her philosophy was to help me work through issues so that I could move forward and learn my own coping mechanisms, but she taught me those tools gently and with love. She put no pressure or time limit on my healing. She merely assured me she'd be with me on the journey, which is exactly the type of support that all long haulers need.

As we talked about present issues, we naturally went back to the derivations of those issues from my past. Michele validated that I had several debilitating illnesses that affected me physically, neurologically, and emotionally. She also helped me see that my response to illness, and to my caregivers, stemmed from deeply ingrained patterns I'd developed as a child. We labored to rewrite those patterns, working toward a time when self-love, and putting my own needs first, would be my natural inclination.

One day I told Michele, "There's another thing I've never really worked through." I'm not sure what made me say it on that particular day. I do remember fidgeting on the couch because I wasn't sure how to bring the subject up. Taking a deep breath, I blurted out, "This guy I kind of dated in college...he was...um, killed, a few years ago." I looked down, picking with my good arm at invisible lint on my jeans. "I mean, I wasn't dating him at the time he died, or anything. I just...um...I just never really dealt with his loss." I explained how I had been at camp at the time Peter was killed, and how that hadn't been the time or place to mourn.

Michele wrote some notes and simply said, "I'm so sorry that happened."

"So...like...maybe I should talk about that." I realized I was stumbling and repeating myself, my face flushed.

"I think it will all come out in due time," Michele said.

Sometimes I dreamed about Peter. In one, I was visiting my freshman dorm room, alone, though I had a sense, in the dream, of Peter's ghost-like presence next to me. There was a soft light in the room, and I was looking around at things as they once were. My lifeguarding shirt and favorite purple shorts were folded neatly on the chair. Two pennies were face up on my desk: one for me, one for Peter. The next morning, I recorded the dream in my journal, ending with, "I took a last look at the room, sighed, and left."

I didn't know how to make sense of these dreams, and I'm not sure I even told Michele about all of them. I had at least 10-12 dreams each night, all so detailed they would take pages to write out. Often, I dreamed in levels, meaning instead of waking up from a dream, I'd slip into another dream in which I would tell someone about the previous one. Michele explained that being conscious of dreaming in this way is called lucid dreaming. A lucid dreamer can sometimes take control of their dreams, and Michele encouraged me to try to change my nightmares into good dreams. Sometimes my dream self could say, "I don't like this," and the dream would either change direction, or I would force myself to wake up. But then I'd just roll over and fall into a new dream. Sometimes the dreams were narrated. I might read an entire book, or read a page of my future writing, or "act out" eight chapters of a story in one hour. I jotted a few of these dreams in my journal, but mostly I just begged my doctors to find a way to stop the nighttime insanity.

The only sleep medication that somewhat worked (meaning it knocked me out but didn't alleviate the dreams and nightmares) was the one that had caused me to "drunk dial" the pizza place and order a salad. Most nights that medicine just put me to sleep, but when I was especially tired, it occasionally made me hallucinate. One night at my mom's house, I called Elizabeth from my phone upstairs to her phone downstairs to tell her that there was an octopus in my bed. She ran upstairs laughing and did not even say I was crazy when I pointed to the puffy billows of my down comforter and explained, matter-of-factly, that they looked like spindly octopus legs slithering towards me. My sister simply patted the puffy parts down, and the "octopus" was gone.

A few months after that incident, I called my mother, again from one phone in the house to another, to tell her that she should come upstairs quickly to see the Russian violinists dancing in my room. Like Elizabeth, my mom played right along. I heard her bound up the stairs, and then saw the light in the hallway as she popped open my bedroom door.

"They're right there," I pointed. "Next to my bed. Do you see them?"

My mother walked toward the foot of my bed. "Here?"

"Yes! Oh, watch out! You're about to bump into one!"

My mom stepped back a few feet. "Here?"

"Yes. Isn't the music pretty?"

"Lovely!" My mom put her arms up as if with a dance partner. She twirled and spun and dipped because she was willing to try anything to make me smile. To make me sleep. To make me well.

Repeatedly, I dreamed that it was the last day of camp, and I hadn't had a chance to water-ski all summer. I'd rush down to the waterfront, only to find that the boats had been put away and I'd missed my chance.

"It's weird that I'm dreaming about actually water-skiing," I told Michele. "I haven't water-skied since before my knee surgery.

Since then, I felt it'd be too risky, and I'm at peace with that. I was totally happy just driving the boat during my last few summers at camp, teaching other people to ski. So, it's weird that I'm not dreaming about driving the boat. Because that's the part I really miss right now."

"Maybe you're missing something else, too," Michele suggested.

"Like being active?"

"Yes," Michele said slowly. "But maybe it's also metaphorical. What could water-skiing symbolize?"

I thought for a minute. "Fun?"

"I think so. Your life has not been fun for a while. You haven't been able to kick back or enjoy the activities that you love." Michele settled back in her chair. "How old are you now?"

I shifted my eyes downward. "I turned twenty-seven in May." With a PICC line in my arm and the realization that I'd been sick for two whole years, I'd spent most of my birthday feeling anxious and depressed. When I blew out the candles, I wished for recovery.

"Twenty-seven," Michele repeated. "This is supposed to be the summer of your life."

I kept my eyes down.

"I bet, subconsciously, you're worried you'll miss it entirely. Just like you missed out on water-skiing in your dream."

"Not even in my subconscious," I muttered. "I am missing it."

"You're missing parts of it now, yes, because you're very sick. But as you get better, you can still have the summer of your life. It doesn't matter when it is." Michele chose her words carefully. She never said, "get back." She was focused on forward movement I couldn't yet appreciate.

"Of course it matters when it is," I replied, hating my bitter tone. "You can't just get your twenties back."

"That's true." Michele squared her shoulders. "But you can metaphorically. You can live a happy, fun, fruitful life, once you are well. That might be in your twenties, or it might be in your thirties. Some people don't learn to have fun until they're my age."

I didn't say anything.

"Do you believe you can still have the summer of your life?" Michele asked softly.

I looked at the ace bandage covering my PICC line. I had to swallow several times before I could speak. "I want to," I finally whispered. "But I'm not sure that I do."

CHAPTER 12

"Slow down, Mom! I want to get there alive."

I don't think my mother heard me. She rolled through a stop sign and swung a hard right at the hospital entrance, swerving as we roared up to the ambulance bay where she slammed the car into park.

"Mom, we can't park here..."

But she was already out of the car, sprinting through the automatic doors, shouting, "Help! My daughter needs help!"

That September afternoon had started like any other when I stayed with my mom. I came downstairs when she arrived home from school, and we made snacks as we talked. She had her usual flatbread with margarine, and I mixed banana slices and peanut butter in a bowl.

"I can't believe you like that," my mom said. "Such a sticky mess."

"Yum!" I put a big glob in my mouth, flipping the spoon over and dragging it across my tongue for affect. "Much better than that cardboard you're eating." I scrunched my nose and ate another spoonful. "How was your day?" My mother had just started her thirtieth year teaching high school English.

"Long, and it was only the second day of school."

"Only 178 more to go," I joked, my mouth full and sticky.

"And to think they already made us have a faculty meeting today."

Suddenly I felt flushed and shaky, like I sometimes did before my blood sugar crashed. Beads of sweat formed on my temples.

"The nerve, keeping us so late on the second afternoon—"

I stood up, feeling lightheaded and dizzy. My blood sugar couldn't be low; I was in the middle of eating. But I felt like I might faint. "I'm sorry to cut you off Mom, but I have to go lie down. Right now."

Alarmed, my mother stood up, too. "What is it? What's wrong?"

"I don't know, I just suddenly really don't feel well."

I stumbled to the edge of the kitchen, holding on to the wall as I took the one step down into the den, then turned to the couch on my right and flung myself over its arm. I was gripped by a searing abdominal pain that made me scream and writhe.

"What? What's wrong?" My mother reached towards me, but I rolled away.

"Oh my God, Mom, it's like someone is stabbing me with a jagged chainsaw."

"What? Where? Is it your stomach?"

I gasped for breath, clutching the right side of my abdomen. "Right...here...below my...rib cage."

"Maybe it's your appendix!"

"No, the appendix is lower." I moved my hand down on my abdomen to show where the appendix is. "This is up here." I rubbed the area below my rib cage. I felt like my insides were being sliced into little pieces. I threw myself off the couch onto the beige carpet, trying to get away from the pain. "Please Mom, make it stop. Make it stop!"

"Okay, okay. You're okay. Here, just try to sit up." My mom crouched over me, trying to pull me upright.

"No! That hurts more!" I thrashed on the floor, kicking my legs from side to side.

"Let's call the doctor. What's the number? Do you know the number?"

Sucking in my breath to hold in the pain, I slowly called out Dr. Raxlen's number as my mom dashed into the kitchen to get her phone. She waved her free hand, trying to shush my moaning so she could hear. She walked away into another part of the house for what felt like an unbearably long time, then finally ran back into the den. "I talked to Natalie. She said to take you to the E.R."

Panting, I tried to pull myself up on the couch, but slid back down in pain. "Can you go get my purse? It's on my bedroom floor. We're going to need my insurance card and medication list."

My mother ran off, taking the stairs two at a time. She raced back through the den with my bag in hand and flung open the door to the garage. "Oh no. Oh no!"

"What?"

"The car's not here. Oh my God, I forgot, Elizabeth has the car. She went to Mackenzie's house." Elizabeth had just gotten her license, and borrowed my mother's car whenever she could to go to a friend's house.

Pain and fear seized me again. I pushed them aside to say, as calmly as I could, "Okay, well Mackenzie only lives five minutes away. Call Elizabeth and tell her to come right home."

For an excruciating five or maybe even ten minutes, I thrashed and howled while my mother paced in front of me, wringing her hands and peering out the window. "She'll be here any minute," she kept saying.

Finally, we heard the engine in the garage and car doors slam. Elizabeth and Mackenzie tumbled into the house. They both stopped short when they saw me. Mackenzie's eyes grew wide. She backed away, as if whatever I had might be catching. "Oh my God, Jen."

My mom grabbed the keys out of Elizabeth's hands. "Give Jen your flip flops. Help me get her into the car."

I screamed as my mother drove. When we got to a crucial turn at the edge of town, she said, "Maybe I should take you to a hospital in Hartford." If we turned right, we could get on the highway and be there in twenty minutes. But I couldn't hold out that long.

"No," I whimpered. "It hurts too much. Just go to the local one." Another hospital was a few blocks away. It didn't have as good of a reputation, but this was an emergency. How bad could it really be?

After my mom slammed the car into park in the ambulance bay of the closer hospital, I stumbled after her into the E.R., hunched over at almost a ninety-degree angle.

The triage nurse sat us in office chairs across from her desk, as if we were here to open a bank account or discuss our taxes. I clutched my abdomen as I rocked back and forth on the seat.

"Insurance card?"

I reached into my purse and handed the nurse my insurance card, my license, and my medication list. "Here, everything you need is right here. Can I please just see a doctor? I'm in so much pain. My mom can go over all this stuff with you."

The nurse peered at me over her wire rim glasses, sizing me up. "On a scale of one to ten, how bad is the pain?"

"Eleven!" I hugged myself harder. "Please, can't you just get a doctor?"

The nurse sighed. "I have to assess the situation first."

"What's to assess? I feel like I'm being stabbed in the gut. Look, I have a PICC line in." I showed her my left arm. "I'm afraid it might be related to that."

"Why do you have a PICC line?"

"IV antibiotics for late-stage neurological Lyme Disease."

The nurse raised her eyebrows. I realized this might be one of the hospitals that followed IDSA protocols and didn't approve of the use of long-term antibiotics. I did not have it in me to fight about my Lyme right now. I needed my acute issue treated, stat.

My mother chimed in, "Look, she's really in pain. Please can't we just get her to a doctor?"

The nurse sighed again. "Ma'am, I'm just doing my job."

Holding my head in my hands, I started sobbing. The nurse gave me an exasperated glare.

I screeched, "It hurts. It hurts. It hurts so much." *Dear God, I am screaming in their faces and still no one hears me. Please help me. I don't want to die.*

Finally, I was brought to an exam room, but still there was no doctor in sight.

"Can't you give her something for the pain?" My mother pleaded with whoever was in the room, someone in pink scrubs.

"We can't give her anything until a doctor sees her."

"Then, please get a doctor," my mother cried.

"They're all busy with other patients," the woman replied. "There are several people in more serious condition than your daughter."

I grabbed my mother's arm. "Oh my God, Mom, I can't take the pain. Please do something." It felt like whatever I'd been stabbed with was now stuck in my stomach, cutting deeper each time I moved or breathed.

My mother brushed my hair off my sweaty forehead. "She said they can't give you anything until the doctor comes."

"That's not how it worked on *E. R.* People came in screaming and Dr. Ross immediately ordered a liter of Lidocaine."

The sides of my mother's mouth twitched in what would have been a smile if this were a different situation. She continued to rub her hand across my forehead. "This isn't TV. George Clooney isn't going to walk in here."

"Believe me, I know. He would never leave me lying here in pain."

"We should have gone to the other hospital."

I knew my mother was right, but I was too distressed for should-haves. I whined, "Just get the pain out of me. Get it out of me!"

The woman in pink scrubs turned around in alarm. "Are you pregnant?"

"Are you kidding me? No, I'm not pregnant. I'm in pain. My stomach hurts. I don't know what's wrong with me, but I'm definitely not pregnant. I meant get the *pain* out of me. Not a baby."

"Are you sure? Maybe we should do a urine test."

"OH, FOR FUCK'S SAKE!" Instinctively, I sat up, which only made it hurt more. "Look, I've been bedridden for almost two years, okay? Two years. Alone. There is no way I am pregnant. Please go get a doctor!"

The woman hurried out of the room, and miraculously, a doctor appeared.

"What seems to be the problem?" he asked. He was thin and young with cropped dark hair and a few days' worth of stubble. I wondered how long he'd been awake.

Holding my stomach, I told him what had happened. He nodded and looked at my chart, but never at me. Then he pressed on my abdomen. I yelped.

"That hurts?"

"Yes, that hurts! All around that area. The pain has not let up."

"Hmm. Well, let's get an X-ray. A nurse will come in shortly to take you."

"Just try to breathe," my mother soothed as she rubbed my head. "Let's do some Lamaze."

I wanted to laugh, but it hurt too much. "Mom, I really am not pregnant."

"I know. But you're screaming like you're in labor. So maybe labor breathing will help." My mom demonstrated by taking a big inhale and then slowly blowing out her breath in spurts. "Breathe with the pain."

I sucked in my breath each time the pain gripped me, then tried to blow it out slowly. The technique didn't seem to do much since my pain was so constant, but by the time a nurse came to wheel me to X-ray, the intensity had lessened.

"Feeling better?" the nurse asked as she positioned me in front of the X-ray machine.

"The pain has decreased."

"Well, you're still all clammy," she said. "Somethin's definitely cookin'."

What the doctor decided was cooking turned out to be a huge pile of shit.

"I read your X-ray and I see a lot of…um…stool, in your colon," he said to my stomach, refusing to meet my eye.

"I'm not constipated. I have a lot of medical issues, but constipation has never been one of them."

"Well, that's what this is," he said matter-of-factly. "I'm going to send you home with a laxative. That should help. You can follow up with your doctor tomorrow."

"That's not stool," Dr. Raxlen said when I got him on the phone later. "I've got your X-ray in front of me. Those are gallstones."

"Gallstones? Like in my gallbladder?"

"I don't know how he missed this," Dr. Raxlen continued. "These gallstones are huge. The pain you felt was one of them trying to squeeze through the bile duct. Once it did, the pain stopped. Were you eating something fatty?"

"Yes, peanut butter."

"Oh, that'll do it. The gallbladder processes fat. You basically set off an attack."

Vaguely, I remembered that when Dr. Raxlen had offered me the option of the PICC line, he'd mentioned the rare risk of the medicine causing gallstones. "Rare" hadn't seemed a likely scenario, then. I ran my free hand through my hair, twirling it around my finger. "So, what do I do now?"

"I'm going to call in some medication that might shrink the stones. Take that tonight, but then I want you to go see a specialist tomorrow and get an ultrasound. You can't play around with this."

The next day I drove to see a specialist at a hospital near my dad and Janet. "These stones are the size of rolls of duct tape. Your gallbladder needs to come out immediately," he said. He scheduled me for surgery the following morning.

"I'll come," my mom offered.

"It's okay. Janet can take me."

"What about when you wake up from surgery? When you have the shakes and throw up?" My mom had been with me after eye and ACL surgeries. No one knew how to care for me afterwards like she did. Janet would do her best, but my mom was the one who had always held my hand, rubbed my head, and told me it was going to be okay.

Still, all those surgeries had happened when I was younger. I was twenty-seven years old. I felt like I should be able to get through this on my own. "I can handle it," I told my mom. "You have school. You can't take a day off during the first week."

"Of course I can. I'll take a personal day."

I hesitated. I really wanted my mom there. But this just seemed like another problem I was causing.

"Besides," my mom cut into my thoughts, "I have Cubby."

Cubby was a stuffed bear cub that my mom had given me before my first eye surgery. I was only nine years old at the time, so the nurses had let me keep him in the bed with me right up to the operating room doors and had given him back to me when they woke me in recovery. Cubby had been with me for all my surgeries. It started to feel silly bringing a stuffed animal to the hospital as I got older, but he'd become a good luck charm.

"Gotcha there, don't I," my mom said.

I sighed. "Are you sure?"

"I already put Cubby by the door."

I slept on my stomach all night, which was difficult because of the PICC line. I woke up every few minutes either worried that the port had come loose or that a gallbladder attack was about to happen. I prayed each time I awoke. Someone must have heard me because I made it through the night without incident.

In the morning, I infused my antibiotics, then put on a button-down shirt, knowing from experience that I would be too out of it later to pull a regular shirt over my head. I French braided my hair, which would keep it off my face but still allow it to lie flat under the surgical cap. I had both hands tangled behind my head, halfway through the braid, when Janet called up to me, "Jen, please come downstairs."

I dropped my hands. My hair tumbled loose as the braid fell apart. I walked down to the kitchen, where Janet greeted me with a somber face. "Your mom just called. She's been in a car accident. She's fine, but she's going to be late. She'll meet us at the hospital."

My heart started to race. "Is she really okay? How bad was the accident?" I studied Janet's stoic face.

"Just a fender bender. She's fine."

I wanted to believe Janet, but wondered if she was just telling me that because I had to focus on the surgery. She didn't say anything more as we drove to the hospital. Terrible scenarios ran through my head as we checked in, went through pre-op, and waited for the anesthesiologist. The clock on the wall ticked off several hours as we waited, but there was still no sign of my mom.

"She's fine," Janet kept saying.

My mom was still not there by the time they wheeled me into surgery.

"I'm nervous," I told the anesthesiologist.

"That's normal." He fiddled with my IV. "This first dose I'm going to give you is like a glass of wine. You're going to feel great in a few minutes."

"But it's not just about the surgery. My mom got in a car accident and she's not here. I don't know if she's going to be okay…"

The next thing I remember, a nurse was calling my name. "Jennifer…Jennifer…" People rarely called me by my full name, and it felt strange to hear it.

Something else felt different, too. I didn't feel shaky. I didn't feel like I was out of control from the medicine coursing through my body. There was a dull ache in my abdomen, but otherwise, I felt completely calm. In my head, a voice softly said, "You're stronger than you think, Jen Crystal." Maybe it was my own subconscious. Maybe it was God. Maybe it was George Clooney. Whoever it was, I knew, in that moment, that I'd survived the surgery and I was going to survive whatever else was coming, too.

"My mom," I said to the nurse. "Is my mom alright? Is she here?"

"I don't know," the nurse replied. "I'm not sure who your mom is. But someone gave me this and told me to give it to you as soon as you woke up." She held out Cubby.

Only then did I start to cry.

CHAPTER 13

After surgery, I started a new adjunct treatment, Integrative Manual Therapy. This hands-on therapy, up and coming in the physical therapy world, is similar to reiki and massage. At the most basic level, it helps get different systems of the body working correctly and together. It includes cranial-sacral therapy and neurofascial processing. Using light touch, my practitioner was able to relieve tension in my head, open up my lymphatic drainage system, and help my body detox.

As I started feeling better, I craved time with friends. I got to see Kendra and Rachel when I was at my dad and Janet's. My college friend Patrick, a.k.a. Paddy, was living about an hour north of my mom in Great Barrington, Massachusetts. He'd sometimes visit and take me out for drives around town just to give me a change of scenery. One day as my eyes were closed, Paddy said, "Tell me what it's like to drive the ski boat at camp."

My eyes popped open. "What do you mean?"

"I want to hear you describe it, so you can visualize it."

The idea seemed a little silly to me at first, but I decided to play along. "The throttle is in my right hand," I started.

"Put your hand out," Paddy instructed. "Show me."

I raised my hand and pushed it forward exactly as far as I would from my wooden seat in the boat. Instinctively, I wrapped my hand around the imaginary throttle, feeling underneath for the red button I'd push to put it in gear.

"Now what?" Paddy prompted.

"Now I look back and make sure the skier is straight behind me."

"Is she?"

I turned my head and looked through the headrest of the passenger seat. I could see trees and road through the back window. I imagined all of that was the lake, and that a camper was bobbing behind the boat. "Yes. And now I shout to the skier, 'Ready?'"

"READY!" Paddy shouted back.

"HERE WE GO!" In one motion, I turned my head forward and pushed the imaginary throttle forward, exactly as far as I needed to go to get the skier up, and then pulled back slightly to hold the skier at a steady speed.

I opened my eyes. Paddy was grinning. So was I.

Paddy wasn't just trying to get me back to an activity I love, if only in my imagination. He wanted me to see that going forward, the throttle was still in my hand.

Paddy and our other college friends Chris and Pete, with whom I'd studied abroad, visited me at my mom's house to ring in New Year's 2006. For several years after college, my friends and I had celebrated New Year's Eve together, sometimes in New York, sometimes in Boston, one year in Rhode Island. When I was teaching in Colorado, I would fly to Connecticut for the holidays and then join up with my friends for our annual parties. We'd stay up drinking and talking until the wee hours. The next day, we'd hug each other goodbye and resume our normal twenty-something lives in various places around the country and world.

When I got sick, partying, traveling, and staying up late became out of the question for me. New Year's felt like a mockery, because long haulers can't simply resolve to get well with the change of the calendar, the way one might resolve to lose weight or drink less coffee. One thing I could still count on, though, was seeing my friends. They caravanned to Connecticut on New Year's Day to bring the party to me.

"Who wants more sugar-free pudding pie?" I held a serving knife aloft.

Baritone bellows of, "Yes, please," and, "I'll take a big piece right here," echoed around my mother's dining room table.

My mom had come up with the idea of sugar-free pudding pie, which didn't taste half bad. I scooped slices onto my friends' plates.

"Tremendous!" Pete cheered as I handed him his plate. "This is just like Paris."

"There was no pie in Paris, because there was no oven, remember?" Chris reminded him.

When we'd studied abroad, I'd lived in a tiny studio apartment with only a mini-fridge and two small burners as a kitchen. Chris and Pete each had rented rooms in elderly women's apartments, and because they didn't feel comfortable using their kitchens, the three of us made dinner together at my place every night.

"Yeah, but she's still serving us food," Pete replied. "And the desserts are still amazing."

I grinned, remembering how we (or I, really) would cook up large meals, laughing late into the evening, sometimes going out afterwards to explore the Parisian nightlife. Smiling wistfully, I reached across the table to hand Chris his pie.

"Watch the IV cord," he cautioned, seeing my arm hover dangerously close to the candles on the center of the table.

I instinctively pulled my arm away and nestled it against my chest. I had to remind myself that my PICC line, and my illnesses, were working parts of my life. During New Year's visits, it was easy to forget, if only for a day. I always rested for days in advance so that I would have the energy to talk for a few hours of festivities. I would often fall asleep on the couch while my friends talked. Sometimes I joined the conversation with my eyes closed, just because I wanted so badly to be a part of things. I clung to these visits as critical social medicine. During the 2006 celebration, I was able to engage more in conversation, stay up longer, and even play a few board games. I went upstairs to lie down during the afternoon, but when I came back, my friends were still there.

I read aloud some more study abroad stories I'd written, like about the time Chris fell into the Seine. We laughed as hard as we always did when we reminisced about Paris, but then Chris said thoughtfully, "You know, it seems like these stories are almost coming together as chapters."

"Yeah!" Pete exclaimed. "You should write a book! You've always wanted more time to write. And now you have it! You can write this from bed! Even if you can only write one hour a day and sleep the rest of the time, who cares?"

Et voilà: an idea was born.

By the turn of the year, I had been on the PICC line ten months. Though my physical symptoms were improving, the sleep disturbances persisted. Dr. Raxlen decided to send me for a sleep study at the hospital where I'd had my gallbladder removed.

The first doctors I saw at the Sleep Center were Fellows. After reviewing my data from my overnight study and listening to me tell—but maybe not really hearing—about my hallucinogenic dreams, they determined I must have Restless Leg Syndrome.

"But my legs don't twitch. Once in a while they spasm, but we're pretty sure that's from neurological Lyme disease. I'm here because I have nightmares."

"We don't really see anything on the data that can help us with that, though," Fellow One said. I later learned that the study was only looking for Restless Leg Syndrome or sleep apnea and didn't track levels of sleep. Had they evaluated that type of data, Fellows Squared might have seen that I, like many like Lyme patients with neuroinflammation, was likely not getting enough or any delta sleep, the deepest cycle necessary for physiological restoration, and that my REM cycle was probably kicking in too early and too often. Had Lyme been on their radar, they might have seen, as I later learned, that my paroxysmal nocturnal leg movements were not Restless Leg Syndrome, but likely a manifestation of spirochetes attacking the sleep center of the brain. I'd later learn that such an assault can cause a reversal of circadian rhythm, making patients hyper vigilant when they're supposed to be sleeping, and fatigued when they're supposed to be alert.[i]

"There is some hyperactivity in the brain," Fellow Two said.

"My dreams are really, really vivid, not like normal dreams.

---

i   Bransfield, RC. The Assessment and Treatment of Sleep Disorders Associated with Lyme/Tick-Borne Diseases John Drulle Memorial Lecture. 2016. Available at: http://ilads.org/ilads_media/wp-content/plugins/wp-cart-for-digital-products/mask.php. Accessed 22 June 2017.

My Lyme doctor thinks the dreams are caused by the spirochetes being so deeply embedded in my brain."

The Fellows glanced at each other in a way that told me they perhaps didn't know what a spirochete was.

"We want to try you on this medicine for Restless Leg Syndrome," Fellow One said. I'd seen a pharmaceutical representative in the waiting room. I wondered if she'd dropped off samples that the Fellows were now trying to hawk. I thought about my visit to the psychiatrist who'd tried to fit my physical symptoms into a box of social anxiety. I thought about my vow to speak up for myself. I thought about all the patients who are silenced or misdiagnosed. I asked to see the director of the sleep center.

Despite impressive credentials as a Board-Certified Sleep Specialist and Insomnia Researcher, Dr. O'Malley was gentle and unassuming. He, like Dr. Taylor and Natalie before him, wanted first and foremost to hear my story. Through rimless glasses, Dr. O'Malley looked me in the eye as I spoke, nodding and sometimes rubbing his right hand over his beard in thought. He seemed particularly interested in the detail and frequency of my dreams.

"So sometimes you travel in these dreams, and you wake up feeling like you've actually been walking around a city?" Dr. O'Malley repeated back what he'd heard me say.

"Yes. My legs are sore. But not restless," I quipped.

"And it sounds like the details of your dreams are very accurate. You're certainly tapping into something…"

Rather than tell me "It's all in your head," Dr. O'Malley was trying to explore what was actually going on in my head and see how he could help quiet my brain. "My goal is to help you get more restorative sleep," he said. "The medication you're on is important. Western medicine helps people in crisis, which you are. But Eastern philosophy gets at the underlying problem. Both are necessary for long-term health. I'm working with a new technology here called neurofeedback, which sort of combines the two schools of thought." He pointed to a padded recliner toward the front of the office. Above it hung a flat screen. "Have you heard of biofeedback?"

Dr. O'Malley explained that biofeedback trains people to improve their own health by learning, through the use of sensors, to control body processes such as heart rate and blood pressure. Neurofeedback works similarly, except on the brain. It uses computer technology to re-train the brain to work efficiently. For me, this would mean re-training my brain to allow itself to sleep.

"The technology is completely non-invasive." Dr. O'Malley moved to the chair and picked up small black sensors. "The computer is simply receiving information from your brain through these, which will be placed on various points on your head, and then stopping the music briefly (which sounds like clicks), allowing your brain to reorient itself to the present moment in which there is nothing else to do but relax."

Intrigued, I walked over to the chair. "Go ahead and sit down, try it out," Dr. O'Malley offered. As I sank into the soft leather, the doctor covered my legs with a blanket.

"I haven't worked with a neurological Lyme patient before," Dr. O'Malley said, "so I can't say for sure that it will help. I can say for sure that it won't hurt."

I appreciated the doctor's honesty. He cleaned the sensors with alcohol and then used a sticky substance to attach them to points on my head and ears. I relaxed as he handed me a pair of ear buds and switched on the flat screen. "You'll hear soft, gentle music, and you'll watch images on the screen that correspond to it. If the images are too much for you, you can simply close your eyes."

"And then what?" I asked as I put the ear buds in.

"Then you just relax. There isn't anything you have to do. Every so often, you'll hear the music skip. Those interruptions are linked to your turbulent brain activity, and they will signal your brain to self-correct."

The music started to play, and while it was as gentle as elevator music, the volume was an assault on my overstimulated brain. I gave out a little yelp. Immediately Dr. O'Malley lowered the volume. "Lower," I kept saying, until the music was barely audible.

"I see how sensitive Lyme makes you to sound," Dr. O'Malley said. "I'm glad you spoke up. Keep doing that for whatever you need."

We were both learning.

For about half an hour, the music hummed in the background while kaleidoscope-style images swirled on the screen. I watched the slower ones but closed my eyes as soon as the visual impact became too much. Frequently, I heard a click as the music skipped. Towards the end of the session, I got cranky and antsy. My legs and hands were starting to spasm. Over the music, I told Dr. O'Malley what I was experiencing, and he immediately shut off the program. "Your brain is signaling that it's had enough," he said, "and that's totally understandable. It's worked hard for one session, and we have to remember that it's in a compromised state."

After he removed my sensors, Dr. O'Malley showed me a computer graph of my brain wave activity. There was a central vertical line on the screen, with various colored bars moving like waves in and out from the line. "Those bars represent the activity on the left and right sides of your brain," Dr. O'Malley explained. "The ideal graph would show bars sticking close to the center line, with equal activity on both sides." My bars were moving so wildly that they didn't fit on the screen. Sometimes they would all shift left, and then all zoom right. "It's like the two sides of your brain are fighting for control," Dr. O'Malley analyzed. "We've got to train them to work together."

Within a couple weeks of neurofeedback sessions, I started noting some improvement. My dreams and nightmares didn't disappear, but their intensity lowered. The traumatic nightmares still came, but not every single night. When they did, I was able to tune them out upon waking, instead of letting them affect my whole day. The waves on the graph started moving closer together.

Dr. O'Malley had me keep a sleep log to keep track of overall improvement. Charting my sleep over the course of a week versus looking at individual nights helped me see patterns, and see that a night or two of setbacks didn't spell complete disaster. As we talked about "sleep banks" and "sleep deficit," I remembered Dr. Taylor's words, "Savings, not credit card spending." I'd never been good at math, but I was beginning to understand that having energy, or hours of good sleep, stored in the bank was necessary for me to move forward. I needed those savings for days when I had bad nightmares or felt particularly sick.

Little by little, I was learning that chronic illness is not the patient's fault. I hadn't asked the tick to bite me, just as someone with depression doesn't wire their brain and someone with diabetes doesn't instruct their pancreas to malfunction. I saw that we do, however, have some control over the way we handle our illnesses. Dr. O'Malley introduced me to the concept of Cognitive Behavioral Therapy. Simply put, CBT allows people to take control of, and change, thinking and behavior patterns that are negatively impacting them. It was similar to the work Michele and I were doing to help me reframe my emotional reactions to certain situations.

In terms of my sleep disturbances, CBT meant thinking about my own sleep hygiene. I learned that in order for our circadian rhythms to normalize, we need to keep a strict sleep schedule. I started preparing for bed by listening to quiet music, drinking calming tea, and taking a bath at 9:30, and then turning out the lights at 10:00 p.m. Dr. O'Malley taught me simple but often overlooked tricks to quiet the brain, such as making sure my room was completely dark, and using my bed only for sleep; he pointed out that if I tried to read or look at a screen in bed, my brain would associate a restful place with stimulating activities. Other tips included covering the clock so I wouldn't watch the hours pass, and getting up out of bed when I couldn't sleep, so that my brain would stop associating the bed with insomnia. I started to think about my behaviors, and slowly integrated better ones. As Paddy said one day, "Good habits are just as easy to form as bad ones. It just takes practice."

One day, I laid down for an afternoon nap and actually fell asleep. For so long, I'd been pulling through the afternoons. Suddenly, without fanfare, it just happened. I heard myself snore and felt my body flutter awake.

"I NAPPED!" I exclaimed incredulously to Dr. O'Malley when I saw him for an appointment the next day.

Dr. O'Malley just smiled and nodded in his humble way, placing the sensors on my head. "Now we keep going."

A few days and naps later, I asked Dr. O'Malley for a pen in the middle of a session. "I know we're not supposed to stop the program as it's going, but I have this idea for my book that I just have to write down before I forget."

Dr. O'Malley quickly brought me pen and paper. "We can't stop the writer when she gets her muse," he said with a twinkle in his eye. "Especially if you're writing about Paris. I can't wait to read this book of yours."

After the session, Dr. O'Malley told me that many creative people use neurofeedback to help them hit their "peak performance." Whether a patient's ultimate results are better sleep or better work performance, it's all a result of the brain training itself to get what it needs.

I remembered Elise telling me that my body already had the tools it needed to get well. I needed my antibiotics. I needed my supplements, vitamins, and restricted diet. I needed Integrative Manual Therapy, talks with Michele, and, now, neurofeedback.

And I needed myself, to allow and help all those therapies to work.

CHAPTER 14

"You've come a long way in a year," Dr. Raxlen said at an appointment toward the end of January 2006. "I think it may be time for the PICC line to come out."

As it had so many times before, my right hand instinctively went to my left forearm, covering the mesh sleeve that covered the port that fed to my heart the medicine that was making me better.

I'd dreamed of this day many times. I was tired of having to take a bath because I couldn't put my left arm in the shower. I was tired of having greasy hair, of waiting as many days as I could before asking Janet or my mom to wash it in the sink. I was tired of my hair falling out, which was possibly a side effect of the intense medication, or of poor hygiene. It wasn't coming out in clumps like a chemo patient's, but there was a very thin patch above the left side of my forehead, and piles clogged the sink. It would be nice not to have to infuse every day, to have two free arms.

It would also be really scary.

"The IV antibiotics are helping," I said aloud to Dr. Raxlen. "If we pull the line out now, won't I get worse? I want to keep getting better."

"I want you to as well," Dr. Raxlen replied. "But we can't keep that thing in you forever. We need to see how your body will do without it."

I swallowed hard.

"It will be a bit of a trial. You may have a couple rough weeks. But you've been holding steady for so long now that I suspect you will level back out. We'll also get you going on oral antibiotics right away, so it's not like your body won't be getting the medicine anymore. We just need to see if it can handle taking things down a notch."

Slowly, I took my right hand off the port. If I wanted any chance of getting my old identity back, I couldn't do it with an IV in my arm.

I made an appointment to get the line out on February 9th. In less than two weeks, my arm would be free.

But would I?

On the night of January 30th, I had the following dream:

> *I was at camp, walking along the beach by the lake. The sand was fine and white, much softer than it really is, and the beach was covered in beautiful blue opals. Somehow, I knew in the dream that the jewels were not sapphires or any other kind of blue stones; they were specifically opals. As I walked, day slipped into night. Suddenly, I was up in the sky, flying above the beach of opals, with Peter. Both of us had our arms stretched wide like wings. Peter was behind me, his arms outstretched over mine, his hands entwined in mine—like that scene in Superman when Clark Kent flies with Lois Lane. I was wearing a flowy blue dress and Peter was all dressed up. He was so real—his hands were soft and warm and when I flipped around to look at him his eyes were twinkling and his cheeks were rosy, his smile was just the same as it always was. He was laughing and happy and everything about him felt as close and real as if he were really there—I could even feel his breath. Suddenly we started to fall fast out of the sky. I was really scared and gripped Peter's hands. He whispered, "Hold on." We continued to fall fast, but at the last moment, we slowed down and landed safely.*

I was shaken, in a good way, by how real the dream felt. All my dreams were vivid, but never had someone from my past appeared in such a lucid way. My previous dreams about Peter were just that—*about* him—hazy, mixed-up visions of him created by my own mind. This dream seemed to be *of* him, like he was actually with me.

I read Michele my written record of the dream. I expected a big reaction to the flying part, to the parts about falling fast but landing safely and being told to "hold on," but perhaps she figured all that spoke for itself.

All she said was, "I think you need to find out about blue opals."

"Why? Do you think that part was significant?"

"The type of dream you had is called a visitation dream." Michele rose from her chair and walked to her bookshelf. "Like you said, it's different from foggy dreams of people. Some people believe that in visitation dreams, the person actually comes to you, feeling totally real like Peter did, to deliver some kind of message." Michele scanned her many volumes, stopping at a big purple reference book called *Love is in the Earth: A Kaleidoscope of Crystals.* Her thick silver bracelets jangled as she pulled the book from the shelf. "This is about gemstones." She carried the book back to her chair. "They all have different meanings."

"Like astrological signs?"

"Yes, you could say that. It might be interesting to see what the blue opal symbolizes. It might have something to do with the message of the dream. The message might go beyond the obvious, of holding on through this scary transition."

I was dubious but intrigued.

Michele found the correct page and began to read aloud. "Blue opal ranges in color from blue-white to deep blue. There is also a blue jelly-type opal that has recently been found in Canada."[i]

"The ones on the beach were deep blue," I said. "Or maybe the jelly-type, because they were a little swirly. Not totally solid in color."

Michele kept reading. "The blue opal can be used to stimulate communication skills and to assist one in voicing thoughts and information which one has not been courageous enough to voice in the past. It provides one with both the freedom and courage to speak freely, and with the wisdom to recognize those with whom

---

i   Guilbault, Melody and Julianne. *Love is in the Earth: A Kaleidoscope of Crystals—The Reference Book Describing the Metaphysical Qualities of the Mineral Kingdom.* Earth Love Publishing House, 1995, p. 455.

this free speech will be accepted."

I sat back. Was an opal going to help me voice my needs? Was it telling that I was able to "voice" my fears to Peter in my dream, allowing him to comfort me as we flew over the beach of opals? Or was all that just happenstance, just a dream?

Michele continued, "It further stimulates creativity and ingenuity in 'connecting' with another, providing for an inner knowledge of the methods and situations which would be most conducive to the alliance."

"Peter," I said aloud. "This has to do with me connecting with him in my dream, because I can't connect with him in real life."

"It certainly seems so." Michele read, "The blue jelly-type opal has been used to enhance one's visioning and to activate the third-eye." Michele put the book down in her lap. "Do you know what the third-eye is?"

I shook my head no.

"In some cultures, it's believed that the third eye is sort of an invisible, central eye, like this." Michele cupped her right hand into a circle and placed it on her forehead, in between her two eyes. "It's said to provide perception beyond ordinary sight."

"Like ESP?"

"That's a good comparison. It's like a portal to a higher consciousness."

My heart was beating fast. My dream of Peter certainly seemed like some sort of "third-eye" experience, as did my previous dreams in which I "saw" things I had never seen in real life that then turned out to be true. I remembered Dr. O'Malley saying, "You're certainly tapping into something…"

"There's more to that paragraph," Michele said. "It also says, 'It seems to provide a clear reflection of that which is of concern and to bring the solutions to the concerns.'"

"Wow," was all I could say.

Michele raised her eyebrows a bit. "The rest of this information is very practical, but it seems fitting for you." She read, "The blue opal can also be used to balance one's metabolism, to assist in the assimilation of iron, and to treat fatigue and hair loss."

I opened my mouth, flabbergasted. "The metabolism thing—I guess that could fit with me because of my hypoglycemia. I'm not anemic. But fatigue and hair loss? Are you kidding me?" Michele held out the book to me. "See for yourself. You can't make this stuff up."

I read the words over and over. Then I noticed the bottom line: "Vibrates to the numbers 3 and 9." I looked up at Michele. "What does that mean, 'vibrates'?"

"Some people believe that stones send off certain 'vibrations' as healing properties."

That seemed a bit much for me. As a writer, I worked better on the level of straight symbolism.

"Are the numbers 3 or 9 significant to you?" Michele asked.

I thought for a minute. "My PICC line is coming out on February 9th. And Peter's birthday was on the 3rd. I sent his parents a card, actually."

"Have you been in touch with them before?"

"I wrote them a letter after Peter died, and they wrote back, but I didn't keep in touch after that. But because he's been on my mind so much, and I just had this dream, I figured I would reach out."

"Did you tell them about the dream?"

"No, I didn't want to freak them out. I just said I was thinking of him, and them, around his birthday."

Michele smiled. "How nice. Have you heard back from them?"

"No, but this was just a couple days ago. So maybe I will."

Michele raised her glasses on her head and lifted her chin towards the book, now on my lap. "Did you also see what it says at the top of the page?"

Under the heading <u>Blue Opal</u> were the words "Astrological Sign of a Taurus."

My hands shook, making the pages flutter. "Is this stuff real? I mean, this really seems to be describing me. And my situation. And the dream with Peter. And…"

"I think there's only one way to find out," Michele said. "Go get yourself a blue opal."

The PICC line removal was swift and easy. A nurse came to my mom's house carrying a plant. "A gift for your new life," she said. I looked at the little pink buds, hoping that in the weeks to come, we would both flourish.

The nurse and I sat at the kitchen table and in what felt like minutes she slithered the line away from my heart, down the inside of my arm, and out. I didn't feel a thing. I never looked to see if the line was cruddy or bloody. I just let the nurse drop it into a red medical waste box, thanked her for the plant, and smiled as I walked her to the door. For the first time in almost a year, I shut that door with my left hand.

I swung my free arm and ran my right hand over it. With surprising energy, I bounded up the stairs and into the bathroom, stripping off all my clothes. In the shower, I wriggled my arms as the water ran down them both. Lathering soap in the crook of my left elbow, which I hadn't touched in over a year, I let my slippery fingers slowly slide over the soft skin. Then I poured shampoo into my left palm, rubbed my hands together, and raised both arms— my own arms!—to wash my hair. Letting the water cascade over me, I prayed that the clock of my life would start ticking again.

For a few days, my energy matched my excitement. I washed dishes, I talked about plans to swim in the summer, I noted to my mom that the switch to oral antibiotics seemed to be working just fine.

I should have said, "Jinx." It only took about a week for fatigue to once again overwhelm me. Insomnia raged once more. My whole body ached in ways it hadn't in over a year.

"The aches are always the first to go and the first to come back," Natalie reminded me over the phone. "I know you feel awful, but let's give your body a chance to settle out from the transition. I don't think this will last."

Every day I looked at the nurse's plant, willing it not to die. I clung to Peter's words, "Hold on," as tightly as I'd clung to his hands in the dream.

Michele had photocopied for me the pages about blue opals. As I lay in bed, I re-read them. Now that my fatigue and hypoglycemia were once again raging, getting a blue opal felt more pressing. I pictured a silver ring with a curved setting holding a dark blue opal. Elizabeth helped me research online jewelers. I didn't tell her the content of my dreams, but somehow my sister understood the importance of this sudden, albeit strange, need for a blue opal ring. She must have shown me a hundred options. Finally, we came across a thin silver ring that had the curved setting I'd imagined. In it sat an oval opal, dark but jelly-like, which looked like it changed hues depending on the light. It also looked exactly like the opals on the beach in the dream. "That's it," I said emphatically.

The ring arrived on February 18th. I decided to wear it on my left ring finger, as a gift of love to myself. No bolts of lightning flashed from the sky as I slipped it on my hand. I wasn't instantly cured. My journal from that day notes that I was feeling particularly achy in my head, neck, and back. With the ring still on, I tossed in bed that night, trying to find the least offensive position. Eventually, I drifted off to sleep. Toward morning, when the sleep medication had worn off, I had the following dream:

> *I was sleeping on my stomach, with my arms out beside me (in the dream, and in actuality). All of a sudden, I could feel someone lying on top of me, also face down, so their torso was on my back and their arms were on top of mine. I knew it was Peter, but I couldn't turn my head around to look at him, so I asked, "Who are you?" He said loudly and clearly, "Peter Mark Westra." It was his voice, his arms, his hands, everything as real as the beach dream.*
>
> *He took his arms off mine and massaged the back of my head, my neck, and my shoulders, played with my hair.*
>
> *After a while, he started to pull away. I knew, in the dream, that our time was running short. I was able to turn around, then, and look at him. He was sitting up, under my bedroom window, silhouetted by the light starting to peek through the curtain. I said, "I miss you."*
>
> *He replied, "Therein lies the pain."*
>
> *"What do you mean?"*
>
> *"You don't have to choose the pain anymore."*
>
> *He started to slip further away.*
>
> *I asked, "Will I see you again?"*
>
> *He replied, "I have to go help other people now."*
>
> *I nodded; I understood this was what he had to do. And then he said, "But even if you don't see me for a while, I'm with you, and all of this is real and true."*

When I awoke, my aches were gone.

Three days later, my mom drove Elizabeth and me to routine dermatologist appointments. The annual check-ups were unremarkable. What I remember about that afternoon was stopping at the mailbox on the way home. As we turned onto our street, my mom pulled up to the curb so I could hop out and get the mail. Placing the pile on my lap as I got back in the car, I absent-mindedly thumbed through the stack of circulars and utility bills. Tucked between two magazines was a small white envelope post marked White Bear Lake, Minnesota: Peter's hometown.

When we got inside, I grabbed the envelope, went straight to my room, and closed the door. Gingerly, I opened the envelope. Onto my bed tumbled a letter from Peter's mother Mary, a photo, and a button, the type you might see with slogans or smiley faces pinned to a backpack. The smiling face on this one was Peter's, rosy-cheeked as he often was, wearing a navy and gold ski hat. Below his face were the words "Peter Westra Memorial Sprints." In the letter, Mary explained that each year Peter's high school cross country ski team, which he'd helped found, hosted a race in his honor. The photo was of Peter's family at the most recent race.

Mary thanked me for writing to them on Peter's birthday. She wondered if she and her husband Mark had met me at the funeral, and of course wondered how I knew Peter at college. Would I be willing to share some stories? She included her email address at the bottom of the page.

The letter fluttered in my trembling hands. I put it down on the soft white comforter of the bed where Peter had, somehow, eased my physical pain through a dream and told me not to choose the pain anymore. I hadn't unpacked what that meant—what any of this meant—but the package from Peter's mother suddenly made it all very, very real.

The only people I told about the dreams, and about this new correspondence, were Michele and Paddy. The dreams especially felt very personal, so I protected them as sacred. On the other hand, I knew the intensity of what I was experiencing was too much to handle by myself. Paddy had had some "other-worldly" experiences following his brother Tim's death, and there were many times when he felt connected to Tim in his current life.

"I'm speechless," Paddy wrote after I emailed him about my

dreams. "As I read, then took the deep breath with you and plunged into the next revelation, I came to a point of simply nodding. Life beyond knowledge, beyond the realm of usual experience – and yet there it is, glistening and as real as the falling snow. I find it more than incredible that [Peter] has returned to you in your dreams – into the wretchedness and horror of your nightmares. What comes across so clearly to me is the sense of softness he conveys in your dreams: his touch, warmth, gentleness, and affection."

Peter's dream presence had helped my physical pain, but it hadn't occurred to me that it had also sweetened the ugliest, scariest part of my journey: the nightmares. If only for a night, Peter had eased my psychological pain, too. And he'd done so in my bed, where I'd laid alone so long, a place where I often wrapped my arms around myself in an effort to get the love and comfort I needed.

I replied to Paddy, "Over the last couple years, one big challenge I've been working on is loving myself completely, despite my faults, despite being sick, even loving the illnesses as part of me. For a while when I thought of Peter I remembered the awkward moments, the times when I thought I said something wrong or dumb. Maybe that's what Peter meant by not choosing the pain anymore. The message he's sending to me is one of only affection and love. I am doing my best to take joy, to remain awed, to leave myself open to all that has been presented to me and all that may come."

What came tangibly were pages of writing. Not just from my own hand as I typed my Paris stories, but from Peter's mother Mary, who happened to be in the middle of writing a book about Peter. I emailed her soon after receiving her letter, and we started a steady correspondence, learning about each other's lives and interests, and of course trading Peter stories. Within a few weeks, Mary sent me the first chapter of her manuscript. Reading it, I learned about Peter as a child, about his family, about the unthinkable pain they went through after his murder. I poured over Mary's words, craving more. She promised to send additional chapters, but she had the sense to pace herself in terms of how much and how often she shared, and in terms of absorbing my response to her work. She understood how overwhelming grief could be.

Mary wasn't just a writer; she was also a former French teacher.

In exchange for sending me her work, she was eager to read the anecdotes I'd written about studying in Paris, helping me shape them into complete chapters. There was no question in my mind that Mary and I had come into each other's lives at exactly the right time.

I wrote to Paddy, "I'm enjoying emailing with Peter's parents, and am open to whatever this communication will bring. I like that Peter and I started over email and now it seems to have come full circle."

"There is a word for this, isn't there?" Paddy replied. "This opening of the heart, where Peter's life lives. I suppose the word is love."

CHAPTER 15

When I saw Dr. Raxlen that April, he said, "It sounds like you had a pretty big wobble after getting the PICC line out, but you've really settled out nicely since then. Your aches are gone, and your hair stopped falling out." He paused and looked up. "It looks very nice, by the way."

Laughing, I ran my left hand through my thickening hair. Since late February, I'd had pretty consistent energy in the mornings. I could run errands, go to appointments, or spend time on the computer. I could read short articles and write full chapters.

"I'd say you're in remission," Dr. Raxlen declared, putting his pen down on my file.

I grinned, immediately sensing both an expansion and a settling in my chest. I glanced at the trees outside the open office window, which were beginning to show small pink buds. A gentle breeze carried the scent of spring. Like the promise of longer, warmer days ahead, I, too, was coming back to life.

I started physical therapy. After a couple months, I could ride a stationary bike or work out on an elliptical machine for twelve minutes. I paced my appointments and my writing with naps every afternoon. At night, I started having dreams of feelings I remembered from my past life: the euphoria of being in love, the joy of teaching, the exhilaration of skiing, even the giddiness of being drunk.

Encouraged by my progress, I was itching to move along. Dr. Raxlen's declaration of remission got me thinking about a budding vision of mine: moving to Burlington, Vermont, the East Coast version of Boulder, Colorado. I knew I couldn't go back to the life I'd left out West. Colorado was too far from doctors and family, and too high in altitude for my babesiosis. Besides, I wasn't well enough to ski instruct. But I thought I might be able to re-create the Colorado lifestyle in New England. Even though I couldn't keep up with the teaching schedule I once had, I wondered if I might be able to find a writing job that I could handle.

One night in early fall while at my dad and stepmom's, I nonchalantly told them, "While you were gone, I found a job and a potential place to live." They had gone to visit Alaina at college, and during that time my plans for a new life had suddenly taken shape.

My dad stopped his fork mid-air, rice falling onto his plate. "How much?!" he quipped, his usual phrase when he is surprised, instead of "How's that?" or "What?!"

"You know how I got that chapter published in *Abroad View*?" With Mary's editing help, I'd been working steadily on my Paris chapters, and had sent one to a magazine that focused on the study abroad experience. "The editor emailed to say she's looking for an Editorial Assistant for *Abroad View's* sister magazine, *Transitions Abroad*. It's an editing and writing job with flexible hours, that I could do from home!"

"Marvelous!" my dad exclaimed.

Janet looked up with wide eyes. "Does the editor know about your Lyme?"

"No. I don't want to give her a reason to think I can't do the job."

"It certainly sounds like you can do it," my dad said, taking a sip from his wine glass.

"I can work at my own pace, as long as I keep up with reading and responding to the articles coming in." I shifted on the cushion on my chair. "Plus, I figure I can try it out from here, first, to see if it's manageable."

"Now when you say from here first…" my dad trailed off, waiting for me to fill in the blank.

"Well, you know how I've been talking about my dream of moving to Vermont. I think I could continue to recuperate there, while working." In Vermont I would do things at my own pace. It would be much slower than the one I'd kept in college, in Colorado, and at camp—the one that had always been expected of me—but my perspective was shifting.

"You mentioned finding a possible place to live," my dad said, putting a forkful of food in his mouth.

I set my silverware down. "I did an online search to see what's out there, and I couldn't believe what I found. The cost of living is so much cheaper in Vermont. I saw this one place..."

"So, show us!" Janet said. I could see the planning wheels already turning in her head.

I scurried upstairs to retrieve my laptop. While I was gone, my dad and Janet finished eating and cleared the plates. I set my computer in the center of the table. The apartment on my screen was a two-story bungalow with thick wood stairs and walls that reminded me of a ski lodge. Downstairs was a cozy living space and galley kitchen. Upstairs was a bedroom, a bathroom, and a second bedroom that I could use as my office.

My dad guffawed when he saw the price. "Wow, the cost of living really is cheaper there. You couldn't get a cardboard box for that price here."

I told him that it seemed like my earnings from the new job could cover the rent.

"And we'd be glad to help with other living costs," he offered.

I bit my lip. "I wouldn't feel right about that."

My dad pushed back in his chair, folding his arms and resting them on his chest. "But if you think about it, we're already covering those costs here."

Yes, my parents were paying for my specialty foods, but my other food and utilities were just part of the household bills they paid anyway. It would cost more for them to pay for my own staples. The guilt of being twenty-eight and dependent churned in my stomach.

Janet swiftly put a stop to that. "It is what it is. You're in a unique situation. This a great opportunity for you to move forward."

"Thank you," I said, tears of gratitude, relief, joy, and guilt spilling over. "I feel so lucky to have your help. Hopefully I won't need it for too much longer. Once I'm in Vermont, I can start to look for additional jobs. And maybe I'll hear from Disability soon." As part of my appeal process for benefits, I'd been sent to a state-appointed physician who, after a 10-minute physical exam, determined, "Though you may get a little sad sometimes, you are physically well enough to work a full-time job." I'd appealed again and had recently been evaluated by a state-approved psychiatrist. I hadn't received a verdict yet, but I'd heard that the more steps of appeal you went through, the more likely you were to get approved.

I still believed my tenacity could pull me through anything. All three of my parents believed my plan was a good one. Dr. Raxlen and Michele both agreed, saying we could do phone consultations until I next visited Connecticut. Sight unseen, I signed a lease starting mid-November, which gave me a couple months to get used to my new job before I made the move.

And just like that, almost as suddenly as it had begun, my long layover in Lyme land was about to end.

Throughout early fall 2006, I edited articles and responded to pitches for *Transitions Abroad*. My health improved so steadily that Dr. Raxlen decided to take me off antibiotics entirely and put me on just nutritional supplements. One afternoon while having a snack with my mom in her kitchen, she said, "Your eyes look so bright. So alive."

If my life were a movie, this would be the happy ending. Sappy music didn't play, but my friends did come to clap and cheer the finale. My mom threw a big "Back to Life" party at her house. My mom and Elizabeth, my dad and Janet, and my aunt Nancy and uncle Steve were all there; Alaina even made a surprise trip from college. Paddy came from Great Barrington, Pete from New York, and Chris and Elise from D.C.; Sharon and Alix each came from New York; other college friends came from around the country.

"Wow, you look amazing," many of the partygoers told me. "Where have you been hiding that body?" one asked. I could have been put off by such a comment but took it as a nod to the fact that the old, athletic Jen was coming back to the surface. I'd been hidden for so long under cover of illness, like being in a mummy costume that had almost suffocated me. I'd never liked playing dress up as a kid because I didn't like pretending to be someone I wasn't. I didn't like it any better as an adult. I wasn't fond of the person illness had made me become. It felt so liberating to shed the shroud of the most debilitating days, to stand at the center of the party and announce, "I'm back!" In a few weeks' time I would be living my life again, not just remembering it.

A few days before I was to make the move to Vermont—the moving van was scheduled, a new bed and couch were purchased, my old plastic tubs with all my Colorado belongings had come out of the basement, and I'd packed up my rooms at both houses— Natalie called.

"We have a problem," she said. "I'm looking over your recent blood work, and your CD57 test came back low."

"My CD what?" I cradled the phone between my shoulder and chin as I zipped up a duffle bag.

"CD57," Natalie repeated. "It's a relatively new test that measures certain killer cells." She explained that those cells target many bacterial infections, including Lyme, and are a good marker of how active an infection is and how well a body is fighting it. The normal reference range is 60 to 360 cells per microliter of blood; the higher the number, the better. Above 300 is considered remission or inactive infection, whereas below 60 is considered active infection.

"What was my number?" I asked, sensing a tightening in my chest.

"Sixteen."

I felt the blood in my face drain, remembering all too clearly the phone call I'd had three years earlier with the nurse who'd told me I had mono and couldn't go to camp. This couldn't be happening again.

"But I'm doing so well," I stammered. "Dr. Raxlen said I'm in remission."

"I know," Natalie replied. "Which is why this doesn't make a whole lot of sense. Based on your clinical presentation, we'd expect this number to be much, much higher."

I pulled out the chair tucked under the desk and sat on the cushion where I'd done homework as a child. "So, what do I do? I'm supposed to move to Vermont in a couple days."

"This test is very new, and we don't know how reliable it is," Natalie said. "In this case, it doesn't seem like the read we're getting from the test matches what you're actually experiencing. You're still feeling well, right?"

"Great. Better than I have in years."

"Okay. Then I think we should ignore the test and stick to the plan."

"So I can go to Vermont?" I squealed, pressing my left hand to my chest in relief.

"Yes. I think you should go. Just keep us posted and let us know if you run into any trouble when you get there."

PART III

CHAPTER 16

Late fall in Burlington blew by in a blur of reading, writing, and trying. Each morning, I ate breakfast in my cozy kitchen and then padded upstairs in my pajamas to my office, in the days before remote work was the norm. From my flannel-clad perch, I "traveled" to Costa Rica, learned about volunteer opportunities in Latvia, and read about the Gross National Happiness Index in Bhutan. People who heard about my job often said, "Oh, that's so cool! Do you get to travel for it?" I didn't know if I'd ever have the energy to gallivant around other countries like I once had when studying abroad, but traveling in my imagination was good enough for me. I was taking things one step at a time, and settling in Vermont raised my own happiness index exponentially.

I loved my new home. I was grateful to have been able to convalesce with family; not everyone who takes a detour from the life they'd planned, whether due to illness, unemployment, divorce, or other adversity, has that kind of support system. But I relished my reclaimed independence, which I'd taken for granted in Colorado. Now I was thankful that I could eat whatever I wanted, whenever I wanted; that I could nap upstairs or downstairs; that I could keep the lights on or off. Best of all, I could surround myself with my belongings in the whole apartment, not just my room.

My mom, dad, and Janet helped with the actual move, and Kendra flew up for a weekend to help me unpack and settle in. In my new bedroom, I was back under my old comforter from

Colorado, looking out a bedroom window adorned with a swoopy purple curtain I'd visualized when sick. My beloved books were back on my bookshelves. For years, the words of my favorite authors had been buried in tubs in my mom's basement but had stayed in my mind, encouraging me on my darkest days. Now it was time to air them out. To air myself out.

I worked for two to four hours each morning, depending on what else I needed to get done that day. In Colorado, I'd done chores like food shopping without thinking about them, in between teaching and grading and skiing and hanging out with friends. Now I had to parse out my energy between working and daily living, something thousands of chronic illness patients have to manage every day. Later I'd learn about the "spoon theory," coined by a lupus patient who demonstrated her daily energy allotment through a bunch of spoons. For each basic task of living like showering, dressing, or driving, a spoon was taken away. Once the spoons were gone, there were no reserves.[i] Before knowing the term, I was living the "spoonie" life.

Dinner was a task I hadn't thought about in my excitement to move to Vermont. Standing in the kitchen, chopping vegetables, and stirring pots was tiring. My spoons were usually gone before I needed to do the dishes. In the back of my head, I heard Dr. Taylor saying, "Savings, not credit card spending," but aloud I'd say, "What am I supposed to do? Let the dishes pile up?"

In the evening, I sometimes watched light TV or talked on the phone, and sometimes did more work. Because I made my own schedule, it was easy to get sucked in to reading just a few more articles or responding to just a couple more emails. I was paid by the hour, and the more hours I put in, the more money I could put toward the expenses my dad and Janet were covering. They weren't explicitly putting pressure on me to lower those expenses, but I put plenty of pressure on myself. I posted ads for tutoring, I emailed three local colleges to see if they needed help at their writing centers, and I inquired if the local newspaper needed a freelance reporter. No one had gotten back to me yet.

I was attempting to connect with my new community. One

---

i   https://butyoudontlooksick.com/articles/written-by-christine/the-spoon-theory/

night, I went to a birthday party for a college acquaintance where I bumped into a couple who I'd probably last seen across a beer pong table. Now they were married and had a baby in tow. "What have you been up to?" the woman asked. The baby giggled and stuck her foot in her father's beer.

It was such a simple question, yet I wasn't sure how to answer. The only people I'd socialized with during my convalescence were friends who knew my situation well. I hadn't thought about how I wanted to present my narrative to new people. The summer I was at Bread Loaf, I had told everyone around me that I was sick. In this new life, I didn't want to be identified that way.

I started with the present. "I just moved here. I'm working for *Transitions Abroad* magazine." The man asked where I'd moved from.

"Connecticut."

"What were you doing there?"

I suppose I could have said, truthfully, that I was writing and tutoring, but that wasn't what came to mind. Because illness had been central to my world for so long, I couldn't help spilling it into this new world that didn't involve illness, a world that had once been my nucleus but that I'd been distant from for the last few years. Like so many long haulers, I struggled to negotiate the bridge between the "kingdoms" of the well and the sick. Taking a sip from my seltzer, I said, "I was dealing with a serious case of Lyme disease."

"Of what?" The woman leaned in, bending her head slightly. "Sorry, the music is really loud in here."

"Lyme disease," I shouted.

She nodded, jostling the baby on her hip, and repeated what I'd said to her husband. They looked like they were trying to discern if I'd said, "Dealing with Lyme disease" or something that sounded like that but was more familiar, such as "trading commodities" or "studying Japanese" or even "buying new skis."

"Lyme..." The man took a long sip of his drink. "Is that the one where you get a bulls-eye rash? I think my sister had that when she was little."

"Yes! Except not everyone gets or notices the rash, so they might not get diagnosed and treated right away."

"Oh really? Is that what happened to you?"

"Unfortunately. I was undiagnosed for eight years."

"Eight years!" the woman exclaimed as her husband simultaneously shouted an expletive.

"Yeah, it was a rough time." Such a statement hardly summed up the last several years of my life, but a birthday party was not the place to delve into my whole story. This wasn't my "Back to Life" party; it was a gathering for people having a night out amidst their everyday lives of working and playing and raising children. When I'd moved to Colorado, I'd slipped pretty seamlessly into life there. This simple exchange with old acquaintances showed me that it might be harder to slide into Vermont step, but I certainly was going to try.

I introduced myself to a few younger guests who were just a couple years out of college. With drinks in their hands and hardly any makeup on their fresh faces, they looked like the Colorado version of me. In terms of where I was in life, I could relate more to them than to my contemporaries.

Despite not knowing exactly where I fit in, I left the party that night feeling excited to even be among the healthy again. I smiled at the sheer possibility that there were opportunities to explore in this old-but-new world. I planned to join social groups and online dating sites. I would hang out at the bookstore and in coffee shops. I would continue to look for local part-time work. There was a book to write and articles to read. There might even be days on the ski slope!

My family and I had been so busy planning my move that we hadn't talked about the fact that the holidays would fall just a few weeks later. Once I got to Vermont, we all seemed to shift to a mentality of done with illness, back to living normally. I wasn't living normally, but I was living, when for years I'd only been surviving. With the large leap of the move, it was as if we'd swept those bad years away. So instead of staying put for Thanksgiving and the winter holidays, I spent energy traveling back to Connecticut for both.

When I returned, my plans for a grand social life were halted by a work opportunity. The Editor-in-Chief of *Transitions Abroad* asked if I'd like to spearhead a research project for the upcoming issue. It would require me finding out detailed information about hundreds of companies specializing in adventure travel, educational travel, eco-travel, community-based tourism and voluntourism, and then writing up specifics on all of them for a multi-page spread. Because the magazine was on tight deadline, I would need to complete the project by the end of the month.

"This would be a lot of work in a short amount of time," the editor cautioned. "You'd still have your usual editorial duties, too. I know it's a lot to ask, but I also thought you might be interested in picking up more hours."

"No, absolutely." I didn't notice the ironic juxtaposition of my words.

I called travel companies, studied their websites, and dreamed about someday exploring the places they toured. The write-up for each company was a couple of paragraphs. Writing one, five, even ten of these synopses was fun. Writing several hundred was simply too much. But I couldn't slow down. My inbox was overflowing with query letters and article pitches. I racked up hours for my checking account but lost hours from my sleep bank. Other than quick breaks for meals, my afternoon nap, and short excursions to do errands, I worked straight through until my 10:00 bedtime every night. I had learned how to pace myself physically, but not mentally.

I was also reading more of Mary's chapters. She'd begun sending a chapter at a time, always telling me that there was no rush in reading or responding because she knew I was busy with my editorial work and my own writing. But reading Mary's chapters didn't feel like work. Her words were a way for me to reconnect with, and get to know anew, someone I'd cared about. I soaked them up. I was learning more about Peter's childhood and high school years, more about his friendships with people I knew from college, more about what his life was like in the years since we drifted out of touch. Mary sent as many chapters as I requested, trusting that I was pacing myself. But like moving to Vermont, I dove right into Mary's work, not considering the consequences of heading straight to the deep end.

Reading and editing Mary's memoir was my first opportunity to help another writer process through adversity or trauma in writing, something that would later become central to my life's work. I loved it. I learned so much about my own experience through Mary's words. I emailed her, "Your writing speaks to me on so many levels, not just because it's about Peter but because of the way you describe your emotions and feelings and everything you've been through. Illness and loss of a child are apples and oranges but your fears, anxieties, ups and downs, periods of hopelessness, loneliness amidst lots of caring people, need to reassure others even when you're the one going through hell, gratitude for simple blessings, newfound resolve to just *be*—it all resonates deeply with me. Your words are reassuring and I'm learning a lot from you."

After a few months, my intense schedule of working and reading started to take a toll. "I'm feeling more tired again," I emailed Paddy.

"How tired?"

"Like I take a quick break from work, unpack half a box from the pile that's still in my office, and then suddenly get fatigued and have to lie down for an hour."

I didn't realize how neurological fatigue could lead to physical fatigue in Lyme long haulers. In my past life, grading too many papers or spending hours on lesson plans had made me tired, but this was a different type of fatigue. My brain would start to feel full, like it used to in the foggy days when I struggled to even flip through a light magazine. I sometimes mixed up my words or had trouble coming up with the right word mid-sentence. I noticed a few aches creeping back up in my elbows, wrists, and knees.

"But you've felt worse, right?" my hometown friend Sharon asked when I called her to complain.

The fatigue I was feeling was more than the average person would feel after a day of work, but certainly not the bone-crushing, shackled-to-the-bed exhaustion I'd experienced for so many years. I could push through it, at least until the research project was done. I didn't consider this might be the start of a downward slide, and that it was up to me to put the brakes on.

I hadn't sought out any doctors in Vermont before I moved. I knew I'd still be seeing Dr. Raxlen and talking to both him and Michele by phone, so there wasn't an urgent need to find local resources. I was doing well when I arrived, so I hadn't looked for a primary care physician, in the same way I hadn't found one in Colorado until I'd needed it. I didn't really understand what "remission" from Lyme meant, what might cause dormant spirochetes to flare, or what local support I might need if they did.

In January, I finished both the research project and Mary's memoir. I hardly had time to celebrate or relax after the former since I had to get right back to my usual editorial duties. Reading the last pages of Mary's draft didn't bring any relief, either. The final chapter ended with a description of a dream Mary had about Peter, in which he was suddenly standing in their kitchen. "He looks calm and content, confident, as though he's traveled around the globe several times on a trip for both business and for pleasure," she wrote. In the dream, Mary's husband Mark exclaimed, "Look who's come back!"[ii]

But Mary wasn't sure her narrative was complete. She grappled with crafting closure on a story she didn't want to end.

"I think it's time to tell Mary about my dreams," I told Paddy. "Her book ends with a dream of Peter, but she isn't sure if that's a good ending. Maybe she'd want to know about my dreams and have the option of including them?"

"I think it would be smart to tell Mary that you want to write to her about these dreams and ask if she wants you to continue... Let the decision be in her hands," Paddy replied.

I trusted Paddy's advice. Having lost his brother Tim, he knew what it might be like for a bereaved mother to receive the type of dreams I'd had. I explained to Mary that I'd always envisioned telling her my dreams someday in person, but that they felt connected to the last part of her manuscript, so I offered to share them over email if she wanted.

"Yes," she replied. "I'd like to hear them any time, and writing them out is fine."

A week before what would have been Peter's 30th birthday, a year after Mary and I first connected, I wrote out for her one of

ii   Westra, Mary Rondeau. *After the Murder of My Son*. St. Cloud, Minnesota: North Star Press of St. Cloud, Inc., 2010 (212).

the first dreams I'd had about her son many years earlier. It was the dream in which I'd been visiting my freshman dorm room and had a sense that Peter was with me, though I couldn't see him. There had been two pennies on my dorm desk, and I'd known they were there for Peter and me. This dream seemed like a sweet, relatively innocuous start, and I used it as a tester to see how Mary would react.

"I think I'm going to just accept your dreams without comment," she wrote. "They are a gift."

And so I continued, writing out other dreams I'd had *of* Peter, but not necessarily *with* Peter, meaning not any of what Michele had called "visitation" dreams. I sent one a day so as not to overwhelm Mary. She and Mark were about to leave for vacation in Mexico when it came time to tell her the most poignant dreams, the ones I'd had a year earlier that had made such an impact on my recovery and had led me to contact her. She asked me to please keep sending them. Mary seemed to crave the details of my dreams the way I had craved the chapters of her memoir.

I wrote out the "opal dream," the one in which Peter and I were flying over the beach at camp, which was covered in blue opals, and when we'd started to fall fast out of the sky, he'd told me to "hold on." I told Mary that I'd had the dream just before getting my PICC line out, at a scary and uncertain time of my illness. After sending Mary a copy of the reading on blue opals that Michele had given me, I sent her a photo of the blue opal ring on my hand. Then I sent her the lucid visitation dream in which Peter had laid on my back on my bed in Connecticut, massaging away the terrible head and neck pain I felt after having the PICC line removed. The dream in which he'd told me I didn't have to choose the pain anymore. The dream in which he'd told me that he would always be with me.

"OH MY GOD I'M SPEECHLESS," Mary replied. "There are opals EVERYWHERE here. We are surrounded by them." She said that the jewel was a specialty of the region in Mexico they were visiting. Mary said our timing had always been synchronistic; she shared that she'd received my original note to her, a year earlier, after she'd written the passage, "I resolved to trust Peter. His friendships were sincere and he had touched lives in ways I couldn't completely understand…He would stay in touch with those who mattered to him in his own ways."[iii]

Mary said she intended to now include that passage at a different point in her memoir, as well as the story of our correspondence, and a few details from one of my dreams.

I thought about all of what Mary had written to me. I replied, "I thought about what you said, that your story must be about more than just surviving grief. I thought about your perpetual mention [in the book] of the 'living, loving Peter Westra' and think that 'living, loving' is what your story is really about. It's what sets it apart. You're not just writing about surviving grief—you're writing about choosing to live and love more fully in its aftermath."

I intended to do the same.

On the morning of Peter's birthday, February 3rd, I decided to join a gym. My muscles, especially my quads, were atrophying. My left knee ached. Instead of remembering that Lyme bacteria love scar tissue, meaning the pain might have been from an uptick in spirochete activity or inflammation from it, I chided myself for not taking care of that knee the way I had after ACL surgery. I wanted to go skiing or snowshoeing on Peter's birthday as a way to honor him since he'd loved all snow sports, but I knew I didn't have the energy for that. Joining a gym seemed like a good first step.

After breakfast, I drove to a gym about ten minutes from my apartment. The heat inside the building blasted my frozen fingers and cheeks as I stepped inside the doorway.

"Can I help you?" a college-age woman asked.

"I wanted to see about a membership."

She pulled out some glossy pamphlets that showed different options from monthly to yearly memberships. The longer you signed up for, the less you paid, but I was wary of making a long-term commitment when I didn't even know how this one day would go. I asked about trial memberships.

"We have one-day passes, if you just want to work out today and see if this is a good fit for you."

"Yes, that'd be perfect."

iii   Westra, Mary Rondeau. *After the Murder of My Son*. St. Cloud, Minnesota: North Star Press of St. Cloud, Inc., 2010 (84).

She took me on a tour and then left me in the cardio area. Only a handful of people were there at that mid-morning hour. Most were older men with shiny white sneakers and socks pulled up to their knees, slowly pushing the pedals of stationary bikes. I chose a recumbent bike at the back of the room. I adjusted the seat and settled onto the bike below a mounted television. Two newscasters discussed a series of storms, including a tornado, that had unexpectedly ravaged parts of Florida the night before.

I hit "start" on the bike's monitor and placed my feet on the pedals. I'd worked up to some resistance in physical therapy in Connecticut, but decided to begin with none here, so I could just pedal. Slowly I began to cycle, keeping my eyes on the news but listening only to the sound of my breath. I kept the pace slow and steady, mirroring the older man at the front of the room.

As the photos of demolished houses and crushed cars cut to commercial, my thighs started to feel heavy. Instead of the satisfying burn I used to get after hours of skiing, this was a dull thickness, like my legs were laden with molasses. Trying to pedal through the heaviness, I clicked the clock function on the monitor and was surprised to discover that I'd only been cycling for two minutes and thirteen seconds. Groaning inwardly, I gripped the handlebars at my sides as I pushed harder. I couldn't believe I had let myself get this out of shape in just a few months.

Above me, the Charmin bear danced around on his namesake commercial. I wished I had his energy. When the clock hit three minutes, I felt the thick molasses in my feet and shoulders. At 3:30, it weighted my fingers and forearms. Next my shoulders slumped with a dull pain. I continued to cycle, slower and slower, like a twirling music box dancer running out of batteries. I was determined to get to the five-minute mark. At 4:17 my brain suddenly felt full, the way it did when I read too many articles. I glanced at the clock: 4:32. In Connecticut I'd done twelve minutes on the elliptical and never felt this tired. In Colorado a five-minute bike ride at a much faster rate, with resistance, was merely a warm-up for an hour-long workout. 4:47. *I can do this. I can ride 13 more seconds if it kills me.* My legs slowed until they were barely getting the pedals around, but I pushed on, painstakingly watching the clock move from 4:57, to 4:58, to 4:59. I wanted to cheer when I finally hit

5:00 but was too tired.

I wasn't sure if I even had the stamina to walk out of the gym, but I had to leave before the girl at the front desk saw me and asked why I was departing so soon, before one of the older men made some comment like, "That's it? Hey, even I've got you beat." Grabbing my gear, I shuffled to the exit with my head down, throwing on my coat just as I got to the door. I traipsed to my Jeep.

Later that day, still tired but no longer feeling completely laden with fatigue, I decided to surprise Mary with a phone call. She and Mark had returned from vacation the night before, in time to mark Peter's birthday at home with his favorite chocolate zucchini cake. In our year of emailing, Mary and I had never spoken by phone, nor discussed it as an option, for that matter. But I thought after sharing such intense dreams, it might be nice to actually hear each other's voices.

Mary sounded surprised but happy when I identified myself, saying, "Ohhh…how nice for Peter's birthday!" She asked if I'd done anything to mark the day.

"I joined a gym!" I exclaimed with false enthusiasm. I explained that I would have preferred to take a ski run for Peter but wasn't quite up to that yet.

"But going to the gym feels like something you can do?"

"Yes," I lied. Just a few hours earlier, it *had* felt like something I could do, and I wasn't yet ready to admit the truth. Sheepishly, I told Mary, "I only rode five minutes on a stationary bike," then quickly added, "but it's a start!"

I wanted to sound chipper and upbeat on this difficult day for Mary, but as soon as we hung up, I burst into tears. The tears weren't even really about Peter. They weren't about talking to Mary; it felt nice, and natural, to speak with her by phone. The tears were about the gym failure. They were about how I'd been feeling physically the last couple weeks. I knew I couldn't continue to deny the reality of what was happening to my body.

Sitting back in the kitchen chair, I wiped my eyes, looked around my beloved apartment, and realized with chagrin that there was someone else I needed to call first thing Monday morning.

CHAPTER 17

"What's happened to you, kiddo?" Dr. Raxlen's voice sounded concerned when I got him on the phone. "Natalie said you were doing just fine."

I'd spoken with Natalie in December, when I was doing relatively fine. I'd told her about my job, about the move, about starting to get settled in my new home. "That all sounds great," she'd said. "Just remember we're here if you need us."

I hadn't forgotten, but I may have waited too long. It had been easy to brush off symptoms because I wasn't experiencing them as extremely as I had in the past. But the exhaustion I'd felt at the gym scared me. It forced me to admit that maybe all the symptoms together, and the fact that they weren't abating even though I'd finished both big projects, meant that tick-borne illness was starting to come back.

Dr. Raxlen agreed. "But this doesn't mean it's a full-blown relapse," he said. "These symptoms were bound to come up again with everything you've been doing. You've been under a lot of stress." He said that stress releases cortisol in the body, which lowers immune function. "A little adrenaline here and there can be good. But the chronic stress you've been under is like walking into a minefield of ticks."

I sat back hard against the red recliner. "So, I basically did myself in."

"Well, I wouldn't go that far. There were a lot of factors going on here. Remember you had that low CD57 test before you left."

I remembered that Natalie had said the CD57 was a new test that measures killer cells for Lyme and other infections. She'd said the normal reference range is 60 to 360 cells per microliter of blood, that above 300 is considered remission or inactive infection, whereas below 60 is considered active infection.

"Yes, it was 16," I said.

"Well, the jury is still out on whether that test is accurate, which is why we didn't worry about it because you were doing so well clinically. But it may have truly been a sign of active infection, and the stressors of the move and your job and everything else just gave the spirochetes reason to start replicating like rabbits."

I laughed slightly.

"The thing to do," said Dr. Raxlen, "is to nip this in the bud. Let's get you on some antibiotics and back to feeling good."

Since August, I hadn't been on any pharmaceutical medication, besides the sleep medicine. I had been maintaining my health with diet and nutritional supplements. They had helped support me overall, but there had been no defense against burgeoning bacteria. Dr. Raxlen said he'd call in an antibiotic that would be good for the specific symptoms I was having. Then he added, "All of this reading and research and writing is just too much for you neurologically. Can you take a week or two off to let yourself rest?"

"My boss doesn't know about my Lyme."

"Why not?"

"I didn't want her to think I wasn't capable of doing the job." I drew my feet onto the seat of the recliner, bending my knees against my chest.

"Well, I think you've shown you're more than capable. And having Lyme isn't anything to be ashamed of. It's not like a secret addiction or something you did to yourself. You were bitten by a tick. It could happen to anyone. I think if anything your boss should be impressed that you've been able to do so much while managing this illness."

I knew, rationally, that Dr. Raxlen was right, but I wasn't ready to receive the message. I didn't want to fully accept that this illness had come with me to Vermont, that it was going to flare in periods of stress, that it was, potentially, going to be with me always. I still saw it as baggage that I was forced to drag along, preferring to stuff it in a closet when I could.

The antibiotics caused an intense Herxheimer reaction as they killed off burgeoning Lyme bacteria faster than my body could eliminate them. My aches and pains resolved quickly, but my fatigue worsened, and the sleep disturbances returned. One night I was so tired after doing the dishes that I couldn't stand it. I'm not sure what put me over the edge, if it was exertion at the grocery store or a particularly bad "Herx" day or just a buildup of several hard days and restless nights. My memory of that night is literally blurry. I remember standing in the kitchen, my eyes blurred by tears and the florescent kitchen light that suddenly seemed way too bright. I remember turning to face the living room, putting my hand on the kitchen table for support but not sitting down. Maybe, subconsciously, I felt I needed to be standing, to retain some agency when I picked up the phone and called for help.

I remember blurriness as I dialed the numbers. I don't remember why I specifically decided to call my dad and Janet. They knew I was feeling sick again and that I'd resumed antibiotics, but they didn't know my day-to-day struggles. We talked every Sunday night, as we had since I was a child. We had only ever talked mid-week when something major happened: when I won or lost a Student Council election, when I was deferred from and later accepted to college, when my wallet was stolen at the remnants of the Berlin wall. Maybe I knew my steady and pragmatic father and stepmother could give me the support I needed at that moment. They must have known something was wrong when my number came up on a weeknight, and I must have known I was in bad enough shape to alarm them like that.

"Hello?" Janet's voice was nervous, questioning.

"Hi," I said, my voice cracking.

"What's the matter?"

"I'm fine," I said through sputtering tears. "I mean, I'm not fine, but there's not an emergency. I just…I just…I'm just so tired."

"Okay, let's break it down," Janet said slowly. "What's causing you to be so tired? What's hard for you to do?"

I finally sat down in a chair. "Everything. I can barely keep up with my work and then I can't do anything else. Laundry is hard. Grocery shopping is hard. I'm losing weight."

"Are you…" Janet paused dramatically, "eating?" She lowered her voice, like she was picturing me emaciated, unwashed and unkempt, drooping over the side of the couch.

"Yes. It's not *that* bad. I mean, I'm taking care of myself. I'm eating and drinking and taking my medication and doing everything I'm supposed to do. I'm just so tired."

"Wow, we knew you weren't feeling well, but Dad and I had no idea how much you were really struggling."

I wiped snot on my left sleeve.

"What if Dad and I came up this weekend?" Janet offered.

"Um," I said quietly. "I mean, could you? I know Dad's travel schedule is really hectic."

"Dad's not traveling again until next week, and you need help. Of course we'll come." Her own voice cracking uncharacteristically, Janet added, "I just wish we could get to you sooner."

Thanking Janet, I breathed a sigh of both resignation and relief. Help was on the way.

My dad and Janet were like Energizer bunnies. That weekend they did laundry, stocked groceries, picked up refills at the pharmacy, took out the trash, and generally put my apartment in order for a few days. They already had a plan in place for someone to continue providing that assistance after they left. Janet had hired what she referred to as "Rent-a-Mom," a home aide service. The caregivers mostly worked with the elderly, but Janet had explained to them that I had similar needs, something that is not often understood about the chronically ill, especially when they are young, and particularly when they live alone.

But despite help, I continued to struggle over the subsequent weeks. Knowing I really needed to rest to allow the antibiotics to work, I finally broke down and called my editor. As I hesitantly explained my situation, she stopped me and said, "Oh, I knew you had Lyme. I read your article in the alumni magazine." About a year earlier, I had submitted an essay, "Tick Tock," about my experience with tick-borne illness. I'd forgotten all about the publication, or that my boss had attended the same college as I and would have seen it. "I remembered that piece and have been so amazed with how much work you've been able to do in spite of all you've been through," she said. My mouth hung agape as I tried to process the fact that all along, the editor had known about and even been impressed by the secret I had so desperately been trying to hide.

"Why don't we have you slow down for a couple weeks," she offered. "I'll take care of all new pitches that come in." She didn't sound annoyed, or frustrated, or any of the negative reactions I'd imagined. Instead, she said, "You are a critical part of this operation. I want to work with you through this. Just tell me how I can best help you and respect your needs."

Without the adrenaline rush or whatever it was that was allowing me to just barely be able to work, my body gave in fully, rendering me once again close to bedridden. Despite the fatigue, I had difficulty sleeping, and when I did, the nightmares were back. Without neurofeedback to steady my brain waves, they were undoubtedly erratic once more. One night I called Elise in a panic. "What if I never get well again?"

I was sitting up in bed, tangled in the sheets and kneading them in my hands, when Elise put her mother, Liz, on the phone.

"I'm visiting Elise right now and she told me what you're going through," Liz said. "Did you know that I had Lyme?"

I remembered visiting Elise and Liz at their lake house in Maine on a day off from camp in summer 2000, before I'd known that tick-borne illness was living under my tanned skin. I'd felt on top of the world that summer, directing water-skiing, staying out several nights a week until almost sunrise, flirting at the local dance club with the bartender. I remembered excitedly telling Elise about him as we chatted on her mother's porch. Had I known, then, that a tiny tick had crawled out of the nearby woods and bitten her mother? Had I known how Liz had suffered? Or had it meant little to me until I experienced it myself, as Lyme often does until someone is personally affected?

"I'm sorry," I said to Liz on the phone. "I can't remember if Elise told me. I can't remember much of anything these days. My brain is fried."

"I know exactly what that feels like," Liz soothed.

I started to cry.

"You're really, really sick," Liz consoled as I drew the sheets to my face as tissues. "This is a really serious multi-system infection you have. And you've got co-infections too, which just complicates everything. I know you're on treatment now, which is good, but those Herxheimer reactions can be just awful. You have to remember that it's just a blip, that you will get through it."

"What if I don't?"

"You can't think like that. You have to believe that this medicine is going to make you better. It did before so there's no reason to believe that it won't now."

"But I'm not as sick as I was before, am I? I can't go through that again. I can't." Cradling the phone between my chin and shoulder, I wrapped my arms around myself, rocking side to side.

Liz kept her voice even. In training to become a Presbyterian minister, the future Reverend Elizabeth Walker knew how to deal with people in crisis. "You're already past that stage. You were doing really well for a long time. That hasn't gone away. You haven't lost that gain. This is just the next hiccup, and you've got to get past it."

"Yeah, I was doing well for a while, but then I ruined it. I moved to Vermont, started working too much, read a friend's book which brought up a lot of old memories, got really stressed about everything…"

"This is not your fault," Liz cut in emphatically. "Do not judge yourself like that. Those spirochetes are really smart and tricky. They probably would have come back anyway. It probably had nothing to do with you choosing to live boldly, but even if it did, so what?"

I stopped rocking and looked up. I hadn't considered that despite the challenges, my move had been bold, maybe even brave.

"Wasn't it better to choose life," Liz continued, "than to stay on your parents' couch and wait for your life to pass by?"

I remembered Peter's words in my dream, "You don't have to choose the pain anymore." Maybe I *had* chosen right.

"I believe that the very act of getting up and moving to Vermont has set in motion the factors that will ultimately lead to your healing," Liz said. "Do not turn back from your goal of independence and wholeness."

"Believe me, I don't want to!"

"I know you don't. But you have to remember that in any successful venture there are always downturns, often the sharpest right before the goal is reached. You can do this, Jen. You can survive Lyme disease and its horrors. And not just survive it but thrive in spite of its challenges. I feel certain that many, many years from now, when you look back at the events of your life, you will be telling people that this incredible past and current challenge of Lyme disease, with its complications, was the one marker event that spawned you for the most future blessings."

Later, Liz sent an email reiterating everything she'd said. Years later, I would re-discover that email and wonder, *How could she have known?*

CHAPTER 18

In mid-March, my dad, Janet, and Alaina, who was on spring break from college, came to visit. Since my dad and stepmom's previous visit, I'd grown physically weaker. Deep circles framed sunken eyes on my wan face after a string of exhausted days and restless nights. My dad and Janet could not hide their surprise when they walked in the door that weekend. Behind them, Alaina breezed in as the picture of college life, her hair long and loose; her makeup shiny, her lips tinged with gloss; the top of her left ear adorned with a silver hoop, the same kind I'd worn in college.

I enjoyed catching up with Alaina, finding comfort in her vivacity. But I wasn't well enough to go anywhere or do anything, hardly able to watch a movie with the family. At the end of the weekend, my dad said, "Now, you have an appointment with Dr. Raxlen at the end of the month. Are you still planning on flying to New York?"

Dr. Raxlen had moved his office from Connecticut to Manhattan. My plan was to fly to New York, go to the appointment, and stay with Sharon for a few days.

My mom had recently asked the same question, suggesting that I instead travel to Connecticut with my dad and Janet, stay with her for a couple weeks, and have her take me to the appointment. My immediate reaction had been "no," because I saw going to Connecticut for any extended period as a definite sign of moving backwards.

When my dad asked the question, I was lying on the couch, too tired to sit up. My dad and Janet stood near the dining table, Alaina behind them in the kitchen. Reluctantly, I told them about my mom's idea.

"I think that's a very good idea," Janet said, enunciating each word and nodding her head to prove her point.

"I don't want to leave here." I motioned across the panorama of my apartment.

"It's not leaving," my dad said gently. "It's just for a couple weeks. Like a spring break."

I smiled feebly; if only I could take an actual spring break.

"We can't just leave you here like this," my dad pressed.

I pushed myself up on the cushions. I was too exhausted to argue. "Okay. I'll go."

I called my mom and told her the decision. Janet helped me pack some clothes, my computer and work materials, and my medications. An hour later we were ready to leave. Alaina was still upstairs in the bathroom as my dad and Janet carried luggage out to the car. I called up to her to shut the front door when she came out, saying that it would lock behind her. I didn't want to be the one to physically pull the door shut.

Still, I made myself take a blurry glance around the apartment, snapping a mental picture of my kitchen, the fireplace, my photos and candles, the view out the sliding glass door. I had a sinking feeling I would never see my home again.

It took over six hours to get to my mom's. Snow and traffic slowed our route. Every time we came to a stop, I wanted to get out of the car and run back to Vermont. My head listed side to side. As we drove straight through nap time, my legs bounced against the seat. My dad asked me questions and regaled me with stories, but I couldn't concentrate on any of it. I needed to be prone in a quiet, dark room. I kept pulling the seatbelt away from my chest, trying to break free of restraint, hoping against hope that we would just get there already.

When we finally pulled into my mom's gravel driveway, I was bordering on the same delirium I'd felt almost four years earlier when I'd at last arrived after driving cross-country with mono. There was excitement about camp then, peppered with a little trepidation that I might not make it there because I was sick. Now there was only dread.

I stared at my boots, willing myself to plod one foot in front of the other as my dad, or maybe Janet, or maybe both of them, guided me up the walkway to my mother's house. My mom greeted us at the door and said something about getting me straight to bed. She stood behind me as I stumbled inside and took each painstaking step upstairs, the weight of my legs and the fear of returning to my sickbed pulling me back.

Once in my old room, I crumpled onto the white duvet. Besides the bed, dresser, and desk, the space was as bare as a hospital room. I had taken my photos, diploma, and framed camp emblem to Vermont. The only picture that remained was the print of the Rocky Mountains that my aunt Nancy had given me when I first got sick. The photo still sat on the dresser, perched like a monument to two former lives: the one in Colorado that I had lost, and the one in the sickbed that I was afraid was about to restart.

Waning afternoon sun peeked under the shades of the two windows, but I didn't feel any light. As I lay once again in the sick room from which I'd finally broken free, I couldn't quell the fear that I might be stuck in that bed for the rest of my life.

I sat forward with a sudden urge like I was going to just get up and drop reality.

But I had no gusto. I fell back against the pillows, completely defeated. I glanced at the clock on the nightstand: 4:06 p.m. Only three minutes had passed. I was all too familiar with lying in that bed for hours, the minutes creeping by like days, the days blending into an endless, stagnant hush.

I tried to close my eyes, but only the left would stay shut, a form of facial paralysis I hadn't dealt with since the early days of Lyme. My right eye popped open as if to say, "Let's get up! Let's look at something! Let's play!" The fight in my head was no different than the fight between my brain and my body: wanting so badly to get up and go, but not being able to do so. I flipped onto my stomach, smushing my right eye into the pillow to hold it closed. At least ten different songs played in my head, a new tune to go with every thought I had, until they were all playing over each other under the steady beat of "Relapse! Relapse! Relapse!" When I closed my eyes, I saw my apartment in Vermont, empty. I wanted to throw up, or crawl inside myself and hide. I rolled around the bed in a ball of angst, unable to get up, unable to sleep, unable to get away from myself.

Eventually I rolled back over and peeked at the clock: 5:02. Then 5:05. 5:09. My mother had gone out to run some errands. The house was completely silent except for my screaming brain. When I finally heard my mom come in, I shuffled downstairs. I asked her about her day, nodding bleary-eyed at her responses. She started dinner. I watched her slice raw chicken as I had as a child and during years of illness. I wanted to offer to help but didn't have the strength to chop anything. I wanted to retreat to bed, but somehow couldn't do that, either. I traced my fingers over the squiggly blue pattern on the place mat in front of me. Around and around like a maze with no way out.

We repeated this routine for days, my mom swapping out steak or meatballs for chicken and me adding fever and migraine to my jumpiness and fatigue. One day my mom came home late after grocery shopping, likely tired and hungry. When I came downstairs to greet her, she said, "Look what you look like." My sleep medication was no longer working. I had been awake for days.

I wasn't offended by her comment. I took it as validation that she could see how sick and exhausted I was.

But then she pointed to my big plastic pill box on the counter. "All these pills," she said, "and you're sick again." Her tone was edgy, bordering on angry.

My stomach instinctively tightened like it had in tense situations when I was a child, cueing me to apologize.

"All these pills," my mom repeated, her voice shaking. "And nothing is working."

"They are working. Dr. Raxlen said it's going to take a bit."

My mom slammed two bottles of electrolyte water, which I drank to replenish after nightsweats, next to the pill box. "It's not Lyme," she said.

I gripped the kitchen table for support. "What? How can you say that?"

"People get over Lyme."

146

My heart pounded and my voice shook as I explained that yes, you can get over Lyme if you catch it right away, that if I'd been accurately diagnosed and treated a decade earlier, I would likely be fine. I reminded her that the spirochetes had spent eight years replicating and spreading. That they'd crossed the blood-brain barrier. "Not to mention that my case was complicated by co-infections." But my mom didn't hear me. She just kept repeating, "I don't think it's Lyme. I think something else is wrong."

"It would be great to have something with a quick fix," I agreed. "But Dr. Raxlen is one of the best Lyme doctors in the world. He's a past president of the International Lyme and Associated Diseases Society. He got me better before, and he's going to again."

My mom opened the fridge and started tossing fruits and vegetables inside. "He gives you all this medicine and it's not doing anything. I'm losing patience with this."

I imagine my mom was scared to see her daughter, who she'd wanted so much for, wasting away. Looking back now, I can see how exhausted and frustrated she was in that moment, as is true for many caretakers of chronic illness patients whose recoveries don't follow a linear path. At the time, I was livid.

"You think I want this life?" I shot. "You think I'm not losing patience with this too? I want to be out living my life in Vermont, working, just like I was doing in Colorado. You think I want some illness that keeps flaring up and stopping me from doing that?"

My mom made some sort of *"phfff"* noise. "You worked for two years in Colorado. That was it."

"I didn't choose to get sick, Mom. I didn't say, well that was a fun two years of independence in a place I love. I think I'll go live on my parents' couch now. IT WASN'T A CHOICE."

My mom sucked in her cheek.

"We didn't even know I had Lyme then," I continued. "It took two years just to get it diagnosed, and by that time, I'd had it for *eight years.* So now it flares. That's how chronic Lyme disease works. You just said yourself you can see how tired I look."

"Yeah? So? You're tired. You push through it. You keep working. It's a luxury to be sick."

"I AM working. I'm just taking a few weeks off so I can get

the rest I need. It's not regular fatigue. Don't you know I would push through it if I could?"

My mom made the "*phfff*" noise again.

"I know I've been lucky to be able to take time to get well," I said slowly. "Not every patient has that. I'm grateful for all the help you and my dad and Janet have given me."

My mom nodded, folding the grocery bags.

"But it's not a luxury to be sick," I argued. "Would you say that to a cancer patient?"

"You should see my friend I work with at school," my mom said. "She has cystic fibrosis. She has to do this pounding thing on her chest"—my mom pounded on her own chest like Tarzan— "and take all this medication, but she still comes to work."

"I work too. Not every chronic illness is the same. People have different limitations and capabilities. Don't you understand I'd rather be going to work, that I want to be in Vermont?"

My mom shrugged. "You were there for what, a few months?"

"I still am there! You invited me to rest for a couple weeks before my doctor's appointment, remember? It doesn't mean I'm not going back there."

I'm not sure either one of us believed that.

My memories of the rest of that evening are scattered like shards of glass that come back jagged and piercing: My mom standing in the center of my room, yelling that I'd gotten myself into a severe depression in Vermont and obviously didn't like living there, that lying around resting all day wasn't going to make me better, that I had to get up and do things—me sobbing on the bed—Elise doing breathing exercises with me on the phone, hanging up so I could do them on my own for ten minutes, then calling back—Elise and Sharon, who was at her Master's graduation, somehow talking to each other on the phone, even though I don't think they'd ever met—Sharon trying to talk to my mom on the phone and my mom saying she didn't want any of these histrionics—my mom telling me to stop this and just go to sleep.

I didn't sleep at all. I tried singing myself lullabies. These, of course, got stuck on repeat, and I spent the night listening to "Twinkle, Twinkle Little Star" try to beat out "All the Pretty

Little Horses," with a side player of "Hush Little Baby." My brain raced in overdrive, sending spasms down the nerves of my parked body, jerking me against the bed. The bottoms of my feet burned, another symptom I hadn't experienced in years. I walked to the bathroom to get some towels, which I ran under cold water and then spread over my legs. When eventually I kicked the towels from my damp sheets, they were hot to the touch.

By 4:00 a.m. I was hysterical, screaming for my mother like I did as a child when I was sick or had nightmares. She flew into my room as quickly as she had then. She didn't hurl any of the accusations she had earlier that day. She just hugged me and kissed my head, her nightgown as soft and comforting as it had been when I was a little girl.

"Alright, alright, it's alright," she soothed. "I'm going to make you some chamomile tea." My mother was teaching the next day and had to get up in an hour, but she sat rubbing my head, holding my hand, attempting to calm me like I was once again her baby. Her twenty-eight-year-old baby.

In the morning, I contacted the doctor. "I'm going to call in something really strong to knock you out for the next few nights," he said. "We may have to put you on another antibiotic to get deeper into your cells, but I don't want to do that until you're here for the appointment and we look at your labs and evaluate you. This medicine is just to get you through the sleep crisis. Your body can't heal without proper rest."

That night, I finally drifted into a sleep that was, unbelievably, less restorative than the endless waking hours. A high-speed mash up of dreams started almost immediately, peppered with my old nightmares of rape, sodomy, and stabbing. At one point I was being burned with a torch.

I woke up screaming, only to find that I wasn't really awake; I was simply in another dream, telling someone about the previous one. I tried again and again to wake up for real, even though I'd been so desperate to fall asleep, but could not rouse myself from the nightmares. I dreamed of opening my eyes, of swinging my legs from the bed and walking across the soft carpet, but my body was as still as a corpse.

As I vacillated between consciousness and unconsciousness, I felt blood rushing to the back of my head, the start of what Dr. Raxlen would later tell me was sleep paralysis, when the brain wakes before the body, rendering the body immobile. I sensed the head rush pulling me down, down into the pillows. I tried to force my eyelids open, to force my legs to move, to force myself to breathe. I was certain that if I did not fight, I would never wake up.

At long last my conscious state won out, and my body actually sprung forth from the bed. Landing with a thud on the carpet, I awoke panting. My pajamas were soaked. I shivered as I slowly looked around the room, making sure I really was awake. I untangled my hands from the sheets and gingerly ran them across the carpet, pleased with the palpable feeling of rug burn. Everything I saw was real: the white walls, the morning sun slipping under the cracks of the window shades, the chipped paint on the desk drawer, the curved handles of the dresser.

My eyes landed on the Rocky Mountain photo. Next to it were vials and vials of antibiotics, anti-inflammatories, vitamins, and sleep aids.

I gulped as I stared at them.

How many would it take to end it all?

CHAPTER 19

I don't know how long I lay shivering on the floor. I looked up at the pill bottles looming above me. I could get up and swallow their contents and no one would find me for hours. My mom had already left for school. But I couldn't let her come home to such a scene. And I didn't really want to die.

I dragged my body across the carpet until I got to the dresser. I reached up and let my hands skim the bottles, but instead grabbed the phone. Sharon picked up on the first ring.

"I don't want to die," I said, "but I cannot go on living like this."

"I know you can't, hon. But you have to hold on. You're going to get through this. Something's gotta change, though. You have to call your doctor and tell him how bad it is."

"I have!"

"Then call again. Tell him you need to be hospitalized. Or call an ambulance."

"I don't really need an ambulance. I'm not having a heart attack or anything."

"You may as well be! This is ridiculous. What is it going to take? Do you need to collapse?"

What was it going to take for any of us to take action, especially if my mom was questioning whether I even had Lyme? If I went to a hospital in Hartford, what would they do for me? I'd heard that doctors in the northern part of the state, away from the town of Lyme where the disease was first discovered, fell on the wrong side of the "Lyme Wars." They followed the strict Infectious Disease Society of America (IDSA) guidelines for treating Lyme and believed that any symptoms persisting after a short course of antibiotics must be the result of something else, though they could never pinpoint what the something else was. They claimed chronic Lyme didn't exist, because the panel who'd written the IDSA guidelines was stacked with doctors who took consulting fees from insurance companies that didn't want to pay for long -term antibiotic treatment.[i] Those doctors, their Hippocratic Oath corrupted by a monetary conflict of interest, fed the myth that trickled down to my mom, that is believed by too many caregivers, friends, family members, and even doctors: *People get over Lyme.*

Despite Lyme infecting more people than HIV and breast cancer combined, it held similar early misunderstandings and stigma of the former illness and didn't elicit the immediate concern and understanding offered to patients of the latter. I couldn't imagine a stage four cancer patient showing up at the hospital only to be told, "Well, we gave you a quick round of chemo. If you're still sick, obviously there's something else wrong with you." But that was my reality. I feared that if I went to a hospital in Hartford, they'd lock me up in a psych ward. What if instead of getting help, I got further and further away from the treatment I needed, dismissed as just anxious, depressed, or crazy?

Moving the phone from one ear to the other, I voiced these concerns to Sharon.

"So have your doctor admit you in New York."

"How would I even get there? My mom's at school. She's taking a day off for my appointment in a few days. I think we should just wait until then."

"You could be dead by then!"

It seemed to me that the great irony of Lyme was that it wasn't actually going to kill me; it was going to take me right to the brink of death, but to actually die would be a choice I'd have to make myself.

Eventually I calmed down enough for Sharon to feel comfortable hanging up. When my mom came home that afternoon, she found me draped on the edge of the couch, my right arm hanging down

---

i   www.underourskin.com

to the floor, listlessly grazing the carpet. Tears streamed down my cheeks. My head throbbed, my mind raced, and my body ached at its core. The joint and muscle aches were much better since restarting treatment, but this was—what could I call it? Not pain, not discomfort, but a feeling of disintegration that felt deeper, molecular even. "I think my cells are breaking down," I whispered. I felt like Elliot in *E. T.* when his mother discovers him and his co-dependent ashen alien, and Elliot croaks, "We're sick. I think we're dying."[ii]

My mom had the same look of panic on her face that Elliot's mom did, but this wasn't a movie. She didn't have scientific troopers storming her house in hopes of studying me. She didn't have the guarantee of a happy Hollywood ending. She had only herself, trying to hold down the fort while quietly worrying about her own health. I'd find out later that she'd had a CT scan that very day, to make sure her lymphoma was still in remission. She was heading into the busiest time of the school year. She was likely thinking about Elizabeth, who'd had a tough first year of college. And she was watching her older daughter wither before her eyes. She had only the conflicting information presented to her: those who told her I was a malingerer, or simply anxious and depressed, or sick with some other physical malady that no one could name; my doctor saying my illnesses were real and incredibly difficult to treat; and me, whimpering before her, begging to be believed, begging for help, begging to be put out of my misery. Apologizing for it all.

"I think I need to go to the hospital," I said. "I can't go through another night like this."

My mother wrung her hands, wiping them on her skirt. "Maybe I should call Janet. She's very practical. She'll know what to do."

I sat up slightly, surprised by this suggestion. Usually, I relayed medical information between my parents. My mom went downstairs to make the call. I was too weak to tiptoe to the top of the stairs and listen. Instead, I closed my eyes, imagining myself in a hospital room with IV fluids and nutrients dripping into my arm; monitors covering my body; friends circled around me, holding hands the way my family had gathered around my grandmother's deathbed,

---

ii   Spielberg, S. (Director). (1982). *E.T. the Extra-Terrestrial.* Universal Pictures, Amblin Entertainment.

the palms of our hands pulsing love through each other to her.

"Okay," my mom said a few minutes later, walking back into the room with renewed energy. "Janet thinks we should go to the hospital." She'd suggested one about an hour away. "Janet said they're studying Lyme there. They might have some new ideas, maybe something Dr. Raxlen is overlooking."

I glowered at my mom, hearing only the slight against my doctor, not the brainstorm of adding more heads to the mix.

"I could take you right now," she offered.

I bit my lip. "Don't you think we should ask Dr. Raxlen first? I mean, they might get me started on some totally different protocol. Maybe he knows someone there?"

My mom agreed and brought me the phone.

"I would not go to that hospital," Natalie said sternly. "It's all IDSA doctors."

My eyes widened as I realized that just because the doctors at that hospital were researching Lyme didn't mean they were doing the right kind of research, or that it was funded by companies that believed in my version of the illness. They might have been trying to prove that chronic Lyme didn't exist. That I didn't exist.

"We can admit you in New York if you want," Natalie said, "but I really think the best thing would be to get you in here for your appointment."

"But it's not until next week! I can't wait that long. I can't. Something must be done today." I looked down at my heaving chest.

Natalie put me on hold for a minute while she spoke with someone at the front desk. She came back on the line and said, "Can you be here at 10:00 tomorrow?"

I looked up at my mother, mouthing the message to her. She nodded.

"Yes," I said firmly. "We'll be there."

When my mom and I walked into his office the next day, Dr. Raxlen was clutching his wire-rimmed glasses in his hand, absent-mindedly tapping one of the earpieces against his pursed lips. He pulled the frames away from his mouth like a cigar as he greeted us. "You look like you've been through the wringer," he said to me.

Dr. Raxlen motioned for us to sit. He rolled his chair out from behind his desk and crossed his legs, his glasses now dangling precariously from his hands as he clasped them around his knees.

"I'm having a really hard time," I started. "I've been staying with my mom for a couple weeks, not in my Vermont apartment—"

"Oh, you must feel like you're right back to square one. Here you finally get yourself settled in your own place, get started with your life, and suddenly you're sick again and back with your mom, probably back in the same bed as when you were living there, too, right?"

"Yes." I paused. I glanced nervously at my mother, then said, "And my mom is beginning to wonder whether I even have Lyme." Tears rolled down my cheeks, dripping from my chin like raindrops. I looked up at the doctor. "Do you think there could be something else wrong with me?"

Dr. Raxlen shook his head. "If the symptoms you were telling me about were new, if they were not symptoms I've seen with tick-borne illness, then yes, I'd be worried something else was going on. But these are all symptoms you've dealt with before. Some of the neurological ones are worse, so we'll get a scan to see what's going on in your brain, but everything else is a clear sign of spirochete activity." He looked down at my recent lab work on his desk. "Your CD57 is still low, and your inflammatory markers are high. The proof is in the pudding."

"So, I'm not crazy." Snot sputtered out of my nose.

Dr. Raxlen handed me a tissue. "You're not crazy. Depression and anxiety can be results of tick-borne illness, but they're not the cause."

My mom sat very still. I blew my nose. "I'm worried I did this to myself." I started going over, again, all the signs I hadn't seen and the stressors I'd allowed to build up.

"This flare-up might have happened anyway," Dr. Raxlen said, echoing Elise's mother's words, "even if you were just lying in a hammock on the beach this whole time. Everything is trial and error with this disease. We never know what's going to happen. You were just paddling along and then bam, you went flying over a waterfall."

"I should have seen it coming." I looked down, wadding the tissue into a ball.

"We have to get you past this perseverating. It's like your needle is stuck."

"I know." More tears spilled down my cheeks. "I know it doesn't help. But I can't stop."

"And the constant weeping," Dr. Raxlen said. "I think we need to get you on an SSRI to get your serotonin stabilized." He put his glasses on and wrote out a prescription. "This is a low dose, but it might be just enough to get you out of this rut." He handed me the slip.

Then he turned to my mom. "I get these questions about Lyme from a lot of families who don't understand the disease or are impatient. You're frazzled too, as a caregiver."

The doctor turned to me. "Your mom is not just your mother, but also a person with fears and emotions and limits of her own. You do have Lyme, and other tick-borne disease, and EBV. And this is really hard on everyone involved."

My mom and I quietly absorbed the doctor's words as he began a physical exam. He decided that I would start a second antibiotic to get deeper into my joints and cells; I'd return to my original sleep medication, the hope being that the serotonin would support better rest; and I'd have a SPECT scan of my brain. "The new antibiotics might cause some shakeup," he warned, "but once we get the sleep back on track, I think you'll start to recover."

I asked how long that might take.

"Let's have you come in again in six weeks. I wouldn't go back to Vermont until then."

"Six weeks! That's the middle of May. My mom or my dad and stepmom can't have me for that long."

Dr. Raxlen looked squarely at my mom. "I know this is very stressful, but a parent doesn't just leave a child when they're sick, right?"

My mom shook her head.

Dr. Raxlen swiveled in his chair, turning to rifle through a filing cabinet. As he pulled out a sheet of paper, he said, "Someone created this for me recently. It may help you both understand the trajectory of this relapsing disease." He handed us a drawing of a turtle with numbers on its shell. Each number corresponded to a symptom category of Lyme disease such as neurocognitive, musculoskeletal, and fatigue. The turtle was meandering across the page. At the start, the turtle's shell had ten numbers corresponding to symptoms on it. As it moved along towards the other side of the page, the numbers decreased. The turtle's path moved forward, then circled back in the opposite direction, then turned around again to head forward, then circled back again. With each turn forward, the numbers on its shell decreased.

My mom and I held the paper between us. "Lyme is the turtle disease," Dr. Raxlen said softly. "Slow and steady wins the race." He looked at us both. "There are going to be times when Jen circles back on symptoms. It might seem like she's stuck in a maze, but you can see here that the turtle is actually moving forward, carrying less symptoms overall as it goes." He explained that the symptoms were numbered by the easiest and hardest to get rid of, the first and last to typically leave and come back again. "It's not a linear path. There are going to be times when Jen has to stop and rest and hide out in her shell for a bit."

As we looked at my complex disease charted out so simply, there was a sudden calm between my mom and me. An understanding, in a way neither of us had quite grasped before, that I would be walking this path for a long time, whether I was in Vermont or anywhere else.

Behind Dr. Raxlen, sunlight streamed in the window, splintering around his lab coat, onto his desk, onto the turtle picture. In the haze of that day the image of the light stands out clearly. I remember thinking it looked like a prism. I remember feeling a sliver of hope that the broken fragments of my life might someday piece together into something new, and if I held that something at just the right angle, I might discover something beautiful.

CHAPTER 20

I kept thinking about the word Dr. Raxlen had used: relapsing. A verb, not in the infinitive, but conjugated, still in action. The disease was fluid, not fixed. It would have been nice to lock in the calm feeling at the end of the appointment, just as it would have been nice to lock in remission when I moved to Vermont. But again and again I was learning that my life was not a movie. I was living the action after the happy ending, and that was messy, just as it is for patients of any chronic illness.

Natalie called about a week later with the results of the SPECT scan. "It shows lesions on and inflammation in your brain," she said. "The left side of your brain isn't getting enough oxygen or proper blood flow."

I should have felt scared but was actually relieved because the scan validated that I absolutely, unequivocally had neurological tick-borne disease. This news did mean, though, that the Lyme had traveled deeper into my central nervous system, because earlier scans hadn't shown impairment.

"We're not talking permanent brain damage here," Natalie reassured me. "With intensive treatment, this could turn around. If you were a new patient and I was looking at this scan, I'd recommend IV antibiotics."

"NO."

Dr. Raxlen had suggested this same course at the appointment, and I had adamantly refused. Getting another PICC line would tell me that I was completely back at ground zero. The doctor had agreed to have me try two oral antibiotics together but did caution that we'd need to see what the scan said.

"I know you're opposed to the idea," Natalie said. "I spoke with the doctor, and he said let's see how you do on oral antibiotics for the next six weeks. If you don't improve, we may have no choice but to put you back on IV."

Back. Back. For so long all I'd wanted was to get back to life. Suddenly I hated the word "back." I only wanted to move forward.

The decision to go back on IV would depend on how the medicine worked and what the spirochetes did, and that was out of my control. But I controlled the environment in which those spirochetes lived. I could choose to make it easy or difficult for them to replicate. I needed to put up obstacles for those bugs, and to pave a path for myself like the turtle's: one that might circle back a bit, but not fully return to the starting point, ever again.

I called my editor and explained the situation. She offered to hire a temp to cover me for a month. Part of me winced at losing those wages, but a bigger part of me knew it was a small price to pay to regain my health. My computer sat untouched. I really tried to let my brain rest. The SSRI helped; I noted in my journal that I hadn't cried in days. Picturing myself as a turtle slowly making her way along a maze-like path softened my attitude toward myself and my situation. I wouldn't yell at an actual turtle, especially a disabled one who needed love and help, so why should I chastise myself?

In my journal I wrote:

> *Dear Turtle,*
> *You slept through on your own last night. That's fantastic!*
> *Your body and mind are STARTING to rest and STARTING*
> *to recover.*

For her part, my mom seemed to be absorbing the lessons of the appointment with Dr. Raxlen, too. I overheard her on the phone with a friend, "This is just what happens with this disease. Dr. Raxlen said Jen will always have these flare ups. She's really going to have to be careful with how she takes care of herself going forward so it doesn't get this severe again." I hesitantly started to believe that her Lyme literacy was improving, even spreading.

My dad called every few days to ask if there was any improvement and if I thought the antibiotics were working. It was hard to say, because my symptoms fluctuated over the next couple of weeks. When I was up to it, I took brief calls from friends. Mary sent cards with messages like "Hang on, dear friend—I need you!" I thought about Peter, about the fact that he hadn't had the luxury of choosing life. I thought about my favorite author, Holocaust survivor Gerda Weissmann Klein, and her memoir *All But My Life*.[i] I looked out the window at the same moon Gerda had watched when she was in the camps, and again when she clung to life on the Death March. I remembered how her friend Ilse, dying in Gerda's arms, had made her promise to hold on one more week. Gerda had kept that promise, and a week later had been liberated on her birthday by her future husband.

Along the Death March, Gerda had occupied herself by thinking about what color dress she might wear to a future party. Clad in vermin-ridden rags, she spent hours debating if she'd look better in blue or red. And so as I lay watching the same moon Gerda had watched, I thought about my future in Vermont, about going on dates and the outfits I would wear, about joining a writing group, about getting a local writing job, about sailing on the lake. I thought about my future wedding, which would be outside, under a *chuppah* or canopy covered in tulips. Or maybe the canopy would be covered in roses, but I'd carry the tulips? No, I'd carry a mix of purple, yellow, pink, and white flowers, like the bouquet my aunt Nancy kept by her kitchen sink, and my bridesmaids would carry pale yellow tulips to complement their purple dresses. Maybe the dresses would have green sashes to tie everything together. The ring bearers, flower girls—nieces or nephews of my future husband? Children of my friends?—would sprinkle rose petals to guide my path.

I thought about my current reality, too, about where I would get the best care. With a month to go until my next appointment with Dr. Raxlen, I wanted to take advantage of the time in Connecticut and do integrative manual therapy and neurofeedback and continue talking to Michele. Since most of my practitioners were closer to my dad and Janet's, I decided to shift base there until my next

---

i   Klein, Gerda Weissmann. *All But My Life*. New York: The Noonday Press, 1957.

appointment with Dr. Raxlen.

On my first morning there, I became so overcome with fatigue halfway through taking a shower that I wasn't sure I'd be able to finish washing my hair. I quickly rinsed the shampoo, skipped conditioner, and shut the shower off. Once back in my room, I lay face down on the bed, still wrapped in a towel, until Janet knocked on the door.

"What are you doing, Sweetie?" she said, more of a statement than a question, when she saw me lying prone. "You need to get up and get dressed."

"I can't." I looked up at Janet but didn't lift my head. "I felt okay when I was eating breakfast, but that shower made me so exhausted again."

"Maybe it was too hot. Sometimes I feel a little weak when my shower is too hot." Janet walked a few steps into the room. "Come on, you need to get up. Let's go for a walk."

"A walk?! I can't possibly go for a walk. I'm too tired to get dressed. I just need to lie here."

Janet started rummaging through the closet. "Here's some jeans and a shirt. You don't need to get all *fahputzed*. Just put these on and we can go. It's a beautiful day outside."

My dad and Janet had not been at the appointment with Dr. Raxlen. Their understanding of tick-borne illness, of my need to rest, was not yet expanding as my mother's was. Janet thought that getting me up and moving would help get my body going, maybe get my spirits up. I believe she meant well. It probably scared her as much as it scared my mom to see me just lying there, wondering if or when I'd ever move again.

"I can't go for a walk," I repeated.

"Come on," Janet urged. "Put your clothes on."

Janet left the room. I slathered on some deodorant, skipped the lotion, and looked longingly at the bed as I struggled into my clothes. Twisting my wet hair into a clip, I slipped my feet into my sturdy black moccasins. Their thick tread was perfect for snowy Vermont paths, but the shoes felt ridiculous and heavy as I clomped down the stairs in Connecticut. Janet was waiting for me by the front door. When she opened it, the light seemed blindingly bright.

Janet held my arm as we inched down the walkway and around the cul-de-sac in front of the house. I trudged along, barely moving my feet, feeling lightheaded yet weighted from the movement.

"You know I'm only doing this because I love you, right?" Janet said.

I focused on putting one foot in front of the other. *Left foot/ right foot, the walker moves through the landscape,* I imagined my college Professor John Elder reading aloud from his Introduction to Thoreau's "Walking," the same way I'd envisioned him coaxing me with those words up the hill in front of my college chapel when I'd struggled to climb it two summers earlier. *Right brain/ left brain, sensation and reflection flicker into the complex wholeness of human response.*

Struggling to make it just once around the cul-de-sac, my best human response was to cry.

"Oh sweetie," Janet said, her voice softer than before. She put her arm around me. "I know this is very hard for you." She squeezed my shoulder and suggested we go sit on the back patio. I gladly plopped down in one of the chairs. The sun felt good on my face, but my body buzzed from the movement of the walk.

Janet disappeared inside the house, re-emerging with tissues and a couple bottles of nail polish. "I need to touch up my nails and thought maybe I could give you a pedicure."

My heart, like Janet's voice, softened. "That would be really nice."

Janet sat in a chair opposite mine and set the bottles on the glass table between us. I picked a pale pink color and slid my foot out of my right moccasin and sock, stretching my leg onto to Janet's lap. "Have you been chewing on these?" she joked as she examined my toenails. "Looks like you went after them with a chainsaw."

"My spatial relations have been off since the neurological symptoms flared. I have a hard time gauging where my toenails are in relation to the clippers."

"Let me see if I can fix this mess." Janet put my foot down and went back inside. She came back with a full nail kit and set to work, gingerly trimming what was left of my ragged toenails. When she got to my little toe, my leg suddenly twitched so hard that my foot jerked out of her hand. "I know you're ticklish, but I need you to hold steady," she said.

"It's not because I'm ticklish. It's because my reflexes have gone haywire. That's one of the neurological symptoms I was telling you about. I can't control it."

Janet looked dubious, but when it happened a second and then a third time, a flash of understanding spread across her face. She raised her head and regarded me wide-eyed as if to say, *Wow, maybe these symptoms really are that serious.*

The moment was so important that I didn't even care that my twitching prevented her from actually painting my toenails. No one was going to see them, anyway.

CHAPTER 21

I joined a local Lyme support group near my dad and Janet's. Members validated me by saying things like, "It's not you, it's a bug in your brain" and "You're right, a 99.5-degree fever isn't high, but it still can make you feel awful." Without falling prey to a victim mentality, I began to see how important it was to connect with other Lyme patients who understood exactly what I was going through. We had personal stories to share; we had a collective story that needed to be heard.

I set up weekly appointments with Michele, and thrice-weekly neurofeedback sessions with Dr. O'Malley. I reestablished better sleep hygiene. Michele helped me get back on track with other cognitive behavioral therapy. I limited screen time. I could email for ten minutes or until my brain felt full, whichever came first. Even if I felt good after ten minutes, I had to take a break.

Besides going to appointments and talking briefly on the phone with friends, I was mostly either in bed sleeping or downstairs eating and taking medicine. I was frustrated that my efforts weren't helping more, but Michele reminded me that it wasn't enough just to do cognitive behavioral therapy; there were still infections raging in my body, including EBV, which was probably also flaring. Only medicine, not I, could control when or if those infections got better. "You just have to be patient," Michele said. Even after all these years of being a patient, patience was still not my strong suit. I was tired of waiting.

My dad was, too. Every night he asked how I was feeling. If I responded, "not well" or "it was a rougher day today," he sighed with exasperation and said, "And...Dr. Raxlen?"

"Dr. Raxlen what?"

"What does he say about these symptoms?"

"I'm not going to call him every time my fever goes up or I get a migraine. That's all par for the course. I'm making improvement, but it's not going to be steady."

My dad wanted results. Michele suggested I invite him and Janet in for an appointment to help them understand the nature of chronic illness and the way such illnesses respond to pressure and stress. My mom had previously come for an appointment, and Michele thought it would be useful to discuss with my dad and Janet how the effects of my past impacted my ability to ask for help, my sense of security, and my emotional well-being, especially during times of crisis.

My dad had his own agenda for the appointments. He was still very focused on how and when I would get better, asking if he and Janet were somehow enabling me. He voiced concerns over whether I could or would be a functioning adult. He was still buying into the mentality that many healthy people have about their friends, co-workers, or family members who suddenly become part of the kingdom of the sick, especially when the illness is complex or the prognosis is unclear: if recovery is taking "too long," it must be because of something the patient isn't doing right. This leads to pressure as well as feelings of frustration, invalidation, and isolation for the patient, which only makes the situation worse.

"There's a benchmark for success," Michele told my dad and Janet, reminding them that before I'd gotten sick, I'd lived independently in Colorado, and before that, I'd done just fine in college and on semesters on my own in both Washington, D.C. and Paris. My inability to take care of myself now was because I was too physically ill to do so, not because I didn't know how. My dad and Janet nodded as if they understood, but later, back at home, my dad asked me if I might be better served by a Life Coach than Michele. As a Business Coach himself, this was the model of therapy he understood.

"A Life Coach could help you set goals and figure out what you want to do and how to get there." My dad stood leaning against the kitchen island, his arms crossed. "They could help you move forward. I'm afraid with Michele you might just wallow in the past."

"I know exactly what I want to do and how to achieve those goals," I countered. "I want to return to Vermont, finish writing my book, find local work that I can manage, and establish myself within the community. I just don't have the physical capacity to do so right now." I exhaled, trying to determine how to explain Michele's work in my father's language. "Michele is a very goal-oriented therapist. She's helping me figure out strategies to keep myself healthy once I do get better. She's also helping me cope with the day-to-day stressors of relapse and is helping me to understand how the past impacts my current situation. I'm not going to get stuck."

"I'm just trying to push you to the next step," my dad said.

"I don't need pushing."

"Okay, then I'm trying to pull you in the right direction."

Getting stuck is a fear that plagues many patients and their families, especially in a society that values success in a way that doesn't have time for persistent health issues. Since seeing Dr. Raxlen's turtle image, I believed that I would move forward again, especially now that I was on the right medication and was getting some sleep. But I still wrestled with immense pressure to make that forward movement happen faster. My journal entries vacillated between:

I'm about to be 29 years old, and what do I have to show for it? I'm dependent, unable to care for myself, a child. I'm wrought with guilt, anger, frustration. This week I've worked so hard to truly take care of myself and do everything right and still I was in bed all day yesterday and totally hit a wall just from watching a movie today. What kind of life is this?

And, a week later, on the eve of my birthday:

This year I will be kind to myself. I will take good care of myself. I will lead a more balanced life in Vermont. I will listen to my body, allow myself to rest, and accept my illnesses as part of me.

Just a few weeks earlier, in my "Dear Turtle" entry, I'd only been able to write to myself kindly using the second person. By my birthday I was speaking kindly to myself directly, a sure sign of improvement.

Since I'd transitioned to my dad and stepmom's house, my mom called every afternoon when she got home from school. She'd started reading *Coping with Lyme Disease*[i] by Denise Lang and Kenneth Liegner, another ILADS doctor. Dr. Raxlen had recommended the book because it explained the ins and outs of chronic tick-borne illness, from signs and symptoms, to the politics of testing and diagnosis, to complications with treatment, to the emotional impact of telling a patient, "It's all in your head." The book also talked about the toll Lyme takes on families, so hopefully my mom found validation in her own fears and her own suffering.

"Some of these cases I'm reading about really are awful," she said. "As bad as yours and worse."

Reading this material was improving my mom's Lyme literacy, softening her approach to the illness, and to me. I understood that in April she'd been pushed beyond her limit, as many caretakers are. We were all learning and finding our way through chronic illness.

In mid-May, my dad and Janet attended a day-long symposium on Lyme disease put on by several ILADS doctors and researchers. "I'd really like to go to this event," I'd told them. "But it'd be too much for me to sit through and process. I wonder if you might be willing to go for me and take notes?"

They said they'd be glad to go. At the end of the day, Janet blew into the house in a rush of excitement. "You really have Lyme!" she exclaimed, as if she'd just read definitive bloodwork, as if everything I had been telling her for over a year was suddenly lighting up in her head like a billboard.

"There's no question you've got it," my dad concurred as he stepped into the house behind Janet.

Janet looked at me with wide, bright eyes. "Dad and I heard all these Lyme doctors talk about their research and their patients. We

---

i   Lang, Denise with Liegner, Kenneth, M.D. *Coping with Lyme Disease: A Practical Guide to Dealing with Diagnosis and Treatment*, 3rd Edition. New York: An Owl Book, Henry and Holt Company, 2004.

talked to so many other families. We learned you are doing many of the right things. And that you have to be on this medication many, many months before you even know if it's working."

Right, I wanted to say. *Exactly as Dr. Raxlen has been telling us since last January. Exactly as I've been trying to explain since the relapse.*

Janet's voice softened. "That was good for us to hear because Dad and I had been coming at this from another understanding which was, we now see, none."

I wish the caregivers of every Lyme patient, of every long hauler, could have this "aha" moment. For patients, the fight for understanding, for validation, can be as exhausting as the illness. To have full support from the get-go, the way those with better known and more accepted illnesses receive, would make recovery easier—and, likely, faster.

When we went out to dinner that night, I felt a newfound calm at the table, similar to what I'd felt when my mom and I looked at the turtle image in Dr. Raxlen's office. It seemed like the burner of pressure to move forward had been turned to low, with a new understanding that I would need to simmer for a while and then slowly raise the flame of ambition that still burned within me rather than reignite it at full blast.

Dr. Raxlen had said not to go back to Vermont until I was really well, otherwise I'd just get myself right back in the same mess. He'd put a stake in the ground: if I was not making significant improvement by the end of summer, I'd have to go back on a PICC line. I was making some improvements. I could type for longer periods of time, could finally nap again, and could sometimes walk to the edge of the cul-de-sac and back. But I couldn't yet do physical therapy. My one attempt brought on the heavy molasses feeling and a migraine that lasted for three days after riding just thirty seconds on a stationary bike. The resulting headache and air hunger, feeling like my limbs weren't getting enough oxygen, told Dr. Raxlen that babesiosis was also flaring, so I was back on the "liquid gold" antimalarial medication that looked and tasted like yellow paint.

"Maybe we should increase your appointments to four or five

days a week," Dr. O'Malley suggested. "To give you as much support as we can before you have to go back to Vermont."

His words stopped me cold.

I didn't *have* to go back. I *wanted* to go back.

I discussed the conversation with Paddy. "Maybe Vermont is not the answer right now," he said gently. "Right now, you need consistent care. You need doctors checking in with you constantly, not every six weeks but every few days. You need to see Michele regularly. And you need to be somewhere where all that can happen." Paddy paused. "A number of us have been worried for many years about a pattern we see. No one's saying you don't have Lyme or babesiosis or Epstein-Barr. No one's saying it's all in your head. You absolutely have these physical illnesses. What's worrisome, though, is how you drive yourself into the ground, leaving no margin for error, blowing past red flags until you're flipped over in a ditch, and you can't seem to see that coming until it's too late."

I swallowed hard. I had done that, my whole life, because I was always part of a high-achieving society that defined success by getting into a good school or getting that next promotion. It required burning the candle at both ends, and there was no time to stop. I'd been unwillingly stopped for so long that now I was racing to catch up, but in doing so, I'd put blinders to hazards.

"So, what should I do?" The phone shook in my hands.

"That's not for me to say," Paddy replied. "The only person who can decide what's going to happen next is you. But whatever does happen, know that all your friends are standing by you."

We were both quiet for a moment. Then Paddy said, "Now I want you to visualize something. Close your eyes."

I obliged.

"I want you to picture your green Jeep flipped over in a ditch. Now I want you to picture yourself slowly driving it back up towards the road. You have that image?" He took my silence for assent. "I want you to picture yourself putting your blinker on, slowly merging back onto the road. There's a rest stop up ahead. Can you see it?"

Tears blurred my vision, but I nodded. Maybe this wasn't the time to do what I wanted; maybe this was the time to do what my body needed. The therapies I needed were in Connecticut.

Nervously, I told my parents of the tug between my head and my heart. They of course worried that my leaving Vermont for good would mean I'd be back under one of their roofs indefinitely. But it was my dad who pointed out that the home I'd created in Vermont could be moved to Connecticut.

"Maybe Vermont was too large a leap," Janet said. "Especially now that we know how these illnesses really work. Maybe we should have had you move to your own apartment five minutes down the road instead of five hours away."

I considered this option. Could I gain momentum in suburban Connecticut, a place I hadn't wanted to put down roots, a place I'd insisted was just a stopover until I got back to my life?

Back. Back. There was that word again. If I didn't go back to Vermont, could I still move forward?

My college friend Alix, who'd so gently broken the news of Peter's death to me six years earlier, used that same gentle voice as she kindly but firmly told me over the phone, "You aren't going to go back to the highly active life you once had in Colorado. You aren't going to be staying up late nights and skiing hard core days. But that doesn't mean you can't have a happy life."

I didn't yet have the vocabulary to know that I'd been trying to make my story a restitution narrative, one in which, according to sociologist Arthur Frank, the narrator returns fully to a pre-trauma state. I'd learn this and other terms years later when studying and then teaching Writing to Heal, helping others literally come to terms with their own narratives. At the time of my conversation with Alix, I didn't yet know that mine was to be a quest narrative, one in which the narrator moves forward through a trauma, bringing its changes and lessons along with her into the future.[ii] Regardless, my friend was letting me know that writing such a future was possible. It might be different than the one I'd always imagined, but it could still be bright.

One late afternoon I sat on my dad and Janet's front stoop, my arms wrapped around myself, rocking back and forth as my mind flip-flopped. *Am I on the right path, with Dr. Raxlen, with*

---

ii   Frank AW. *The Wounded Storyteller.* Chicago, IL: University of Chicago Press; 1995.

my protocol? Should I stay in Connecticut? Would it be giving up entirely? I lowered my head and closed my eyes. *Please, just give me some kind of sign of what I'm supposed to do.*

Eventually I stood up and stretched, something I was starting to be able to do without pain or fatigue. I reached my arms up and arched my back, exhaling loudly as I brought my hands down to my sides. Turning, I steadily and deliberately stepped, *left foot/ right foot, left foot/right foot*, until I'd gone about ten paces to the edge of the driveway.

And there, directly in my path, inching along residential suburban Connecticut pavement with no water in sight, was a turtle.

PART IV

CHAPTER 22

Shortly thereafter, a letter came from the State of Connecticut saying that my appeal process for Disability Benefits had made it to the final step: going before a judge.

My state-appointed lawyer reminded me that putting on my best face was not always putting on an honest face. "This judge will see you for only a few minutes," she said. "He has to see what it's like for you on your very worst days. You have to tell him exactly how debilitating your symptoms can be." In this case, doing my best meant allowing myself to show my worst.

I stood before that judge and told him the truth. I started from the first low blood sugar reaction in 1997 and explained exactly how my life, and my illnesses, had unfolded since then. After just a few minutes, he declared, "I've heard enough" in a voice that told me, "Waste no more energy on this. I believe you."

His decision letter was equally validating. He chided the state doctors who had missed my obvious case, praised the doctors who were treating me, and recognized me as a go-getter whose ambition happened to have been halted by a tick. The fight for validation and financial assistance took over two years. Many patients understandably give up by then, never receiving the aid they so desperately need, especially if they live in a state where the debilitating effects of late-stage Lyme disease aren't well known.

I was awarded backpay for the years I hadn't been able to work. The amount was nowhere near what I would have earned during that time had I been healthy, but it was enough to pay off my credit cards and leave a little padding. I would also start to receive a monthly stipend, which would enable me to get my own apartment. It took several months for me to find a place near my dad and Janet, but we were all starting to understand that there is no timeline for chronic illness.

My dad and Janet had gone up to Vermont to get my Jeep, pack up my apartment, and bring my life back to me in boxes. When I at last unpacked those boxes in my new place, I learned why Alaina had been stalling upstairs when we'd left Vermont; she'd been posting inspirational notes on my mirrors. My dad and Janet had found the notes and thrown them in with my things. Post-its with "You've got this!" and "You're beautiful!" and "What's going to be great about today?" greeted me as I unpacked each box. They were exactly what I needed to see as movers brought my furniture into yet another home, one that I hoped would last, at least until I was ready to take another step forward instead of backward.

My mom stocked my freezer with meals so I wouldn't have to expend energy cooking, and my dad and Janet stopped by every few days to assist with household chores. With help, I settled in well to my garden apartment that welcomed lots of sunlight and overlooked a playground.

"Does the noise bother you?" my mom asked.

"Are you kidding? It's like being at camp. There's no better sound than children at play."

The only problem with a garden level apartment was that it attracted ticks. While sitting on my patio one day, a tick crawled onto the page of the magazine I was reading. "Absolutely not," I seethed. "I am finally able to read. No way a tick is going to ruin that again." I slammed the magazine on the table, smushing the tick and then grinding its guts into the ceramic tile for good measure. I'd thought my patio would be safe, since it wasn't near grass and was surrounded only by hydrangeas, and the table and chairs were in the center of the concrete floor.

"Ticks will hang on the edge of low plants," Dr. Raxlen told me. "They're hungry for a meal. Remember that mice and birds carry them, too. It's not just the deer."

After that I boycotted the porch, but the ticks followed me inside. One day I woke up from my nap to find five or six ticks crawling along the low white windowsill in my bedroom. I thought I was going crazy, but I took photos and sent them to people in my Lyme support group, and they confirmed my fears. The group was comprised mostly of parents with school-aged kids. Many of the adults had tick-borne disease themselves, and all their children were sick. Some families described one child going out to play and subsequently missing two years of school; then a second and a third child would be sideswiped in their own backyard. Sometimes they found the tick bites or rashes. Sometimes they didn't. Always, the family's life was in ruins. In addition to physical, emotional, and financial upheaval, one couple had been accused of negligence by school administrators, and the Department of Children and Family Services was threatening to take their bedridden daughter away if they didn't send her back to school.

I called maintenance and frantically told them that I was recovering from tick-borne illness and could not, would not come under re-attack in my own home. They came immediately to spray the bushes that framed my window, as well as the sill itself, and from then on, I kept the windows closed and the AC running. I loved fresh air, but I needed to protect my turf.

I felt slightly more in control of my life, even if that life was hyper-controlled by appointments, medications, timed computer hours, and rest. The two oral antibiotics were relieving my symptoms. Having finished the course of "liquid gold" for babesiosis, I re-started physical therapy, albeit very, very slowly. My physical therapist Cindy was also an integrative manual therapist, so she did neurofascial processing and cranial sacral therapy. Physical exercise began at a micro-level. Cindy gave me a piece of rubber with holes cut out for fingers. I manipulated the material, working to strengthen my hand muscles without making them ache. If they did get too tired, Cindy would give me pen and paper and have me draw the yin-yang sign. I'd trace it over and over. It was indeed a delicate balance, pushing myself enough to move forward, but also knowing when to stop before I crashed.

Eventually I could cycle one minute on the stationary bike without fatigue or headache. I stayed at that one-minute level for a week, then went up to 1:15 the next week, then 1:30, and so on. As with the first time I'd done physical therapy, before moving to Vermont, this progress didn't move at a steady continuum. I sometimes had to cycle fewer minutes than I had previously, and sometimes had to wait a week or two before I could cycle again. Then I'd start over. 1:00, 1:15, 1:30…

Taking care of myself was now my full-time job, and as such, I decided to step down entirely from my position at *Transitions Abroad*. My pride cringed a little at the decision, but I finally understood that it was more important to rack up hours in my sleep and energy accounts than my bank account. My body sighed with relief.

Without editorial work usurping my "spoons," I was able to grocery shop and drive myself to appointments. My life wasn't exactly exciting, but unlike in the past, there was some margin for error. There was even some time for socialization. Weekly, Kendra and Rachel came over for dinner. Friends who happened to be in the area on business, including Heather from Colorado, visited. It didn't bother Heather that I couldn't ski or stay out late like we used to. She was happy just to see me well enough to live on my own. She, like Kendra and Rachel, like Sharon, like Paddy and Elise and other friends, had known me before illness and had known me through it. In Vermont, I'd tried to move to an "after" period. Now I understood that there wasn't a distinct line between being sick and being well. I would probably spend my life bridging those two islands, which was certainly better than drowning in the waters between them. To bridge was to carry myself safely between worlds, on my own two feet.

For my thirtieth birthday, my dad and Janet threw a party at my favorite local restaurant. I wore a new pink dress, a size bigger than I'd worn during the worst of the relapse. The party was in a private side room. "I asked them to keep the music and lighting low, so it would be okay for your brain," my dad whispered to me when I walked in. My mom made sugar free pudding pie for all. Kendra and Rachel, my aunt Nancy and uncle Steve, and a few of my dad and Janet's friends who'd known me since childhood were all there to help celebrate. I didn't have a big community in

Connecticut, but I did have people who supported me, who were willing to come together to mark this milestone—one which, a year earlier, I wasn't sure I'd see.

In the front of the room hung a giant photo of me at age two or three. Whoever took the photo had caught me in a jubilant moment with outstretched arms, clapping my hands together. I'm wearing a white party dress with tiny red dots. My big brown eyes are sparkly, my cheeks pink. My face is the picture of joy and innocence. I'm tilting my head to the left, as if to get a new perspective on something. Later, after eye surgeries, we'd learn that tilting my head was simply my way of adapting to not having binocular vision; my brain made do with what it had.

Standing under that blown-up younger version of myself at my thirtieth birthday party, I attempted to recreate the image. I tipped my head, stretched my arms out in front of me and clasped my hands. I'd lost my innocence but had a new perspective. My body and brain were adapting to what they had: chronic illness that couldn't be repaired, but that could be lived with, and that could even put joy on my face and a twinkle in my eye.

The little girl I'd once been was standing right behind me, cheering me on.

CHAPTER 23

I revised some of the early chapters of my book about Paris and wrote more, finishing a couple chapters a week. I delighted in being able to exercise my creativity, in finding exactly the right words, in receiving feedback from Paddy or Mary that pushed my writing to a new level. Mary diligently read every word, giving edits, and telling me about her own time in Paris, and about time visiting the city with Peter when he was a boy. I loved continuing to learn details of Peter's life, but no longer clung to them. They nourished me in a healthy way, without serving to fill a void. I reacted to Mary's stories with smiles instead of tears, with gratitude instead of longing.

That summer, Mary flew to New York to visit Peter's sister and invited me to meet her for lunch. I took the one-hour train early one morning, not even tiring as I walked up from the platform to meet Mary, who seemed as comfortable as an old friend as we hugged under the Grand Central clock. We walked a few blocks to her daughter's apartment, where we sat and talked until it was time for my train home.

"It was great," I wrote to Paddy later. "Just totally natural, not awkward or intense at all, and my energy level was good. We got lunch, looked at family photo albums, and laughed. There weren't even any tears."

"Well," Paddy replied, "It's good not to cry on your first date."

Actual dating was not something I'd done in many years. I'd considered it in Vermont, but I'd gotten too sick before I'd been able to get back in the game. I hadn't had a boyfriend since Jim in Colorado, and hadn't thought about him, or a relationship, or sex, in the years that I'd had to focus solely on survival. Now the possibility of dating tempted me.

It also terrified me.

Though I was establishing a steady new rhythm to my life, it wasn't "normal" by any healthy person's standards. How would I explain my chronic illnesses to a potential romantic partner? Did I want to? Did I have to?

"It's not like you have an STI," Kendra said. "You don't have to make a big dramatic announcement. Lyme is just a part of who you are, and you have some limitations from it, but there are lots of other parts to you, too."

I tested this theory on some men I met on dating sites. The first few were not matches. One rambled on about the video games he designed featuring Rudolph the Red-Nosed Reindeer. Another bragged about his cooking prowess, but when I asked what he made, he said, "Well I just buy food that's already prepared by the grocery store, and I heat it up on pans." The stories made for good laughs with the girls, and also reminded me that I still knew how to meet people, how to carry on normal conversation—however "normal" was defined here—and still generally knew how to date. When one of the men kissed me goodnight, it was no big deal.

Toward the end of the summer, I met a French guy who was originally from my favorite town of Annecy, at the base of Chamonix, where Chris, Pete, Paddy, my hometown friend Tony, and I had once skied in a blizzard.

"It's fate!" Elise squealed.

The Frenchman turned out not to be my soul mate. His hubris and cynicism outshined his better qualities fairly quickly, so I wasn't sad when he disappeared after a few dates. I was happy to have had the practice, though, and to know that the romantic side of me was reawakening.

I did like practicing French, especially as I was getting deeper into the writing of my book, so I found a French conversation group. I met a friendly couple who were my age, and a lovely woman about a decade older than us who had also studied in Paris years earlier. Single with her own business, this woman inspired me. She didn't fit into cultural norms, but she was living a happy and fulfilling life, meeting new people, stretching her comfort zone for the fun of it.

My new friends were excited to hear about my book. One day in August, I suddenly typed the last paragraph of the last chapter. I wrote how the end of my semester abroad had forced me to let go of Chris and Pete, and of Paris, even though I desperately did not want to. I wrote about how my heart broke and burst as I took the leap into the rest of my life, knowing that our time together would always be with me as I moved forward into the unknown.

As I'd left Paris in 1999, I couldn't have seen how the subsequent nine years would unfold. Sitting at my desk in 2008, I didn't know how the next decade would unfold, either. But my keyboard gave me some agency. Through it, I had the power to jump back to a happier time, to a place that had filled me with enough life and love to carry me through the last decade. The story, going backwards and forwards, was mine to write.

The question after finishing my book was what to do with it. I didn't know much about the publication process. In early fall, Janet heard about a publishing and writing workshop that was being held a few towns away. There, I met a consultant who took interest in my project. "I have an agent friend who sold a France memoir to a major publishing house. Rumor has it they want to do another book about France."

My friends decided my book was going to be a bestseller, my dad thought I'd written the great American novel—"it's a memoir, Dad, not a novel"—and my mom was ready to see me on Oprah. "Not so fast," I told them. "I haven't even spoken with the agent yet."

For her part, the agent thought she'd have an easy sale. "I'll send it to the publishing house," she said after reading the manuscript. "If they say no, I don't know that I'll have the bandwidth to send it elsewhere. But let's see what they say."

The publishing world moved no faster than Lyme treatment, so I was back to waiting. I bided my time volunteering once a week at a Red Cross blood drive. I wanted to dip my toe back into the working world without making a commitment until I knew I could really do it, and I was eager to help others. Volunteering seemed like the perfect first step. If I couldn't physically or neurologically handle the "job," it wasn't going to be the end of the world for me to step down.

In general, I handled my new role just fine. I liked being on the other side of something health-related. Occasionally I needed to cancel because I was too tired, or because I had to go to a doctor's appointment, but this was good practice for me to put my health first. I also got to practice speaking up on behalf of little things that wouldn't have bothered me in my healthier days but were a big deal to me now. One day I had to ask the head nurse to turn the music down, because the loud, heavy beats were grating on my brain, making it impossible for me to concentrate on checking people in. She gave me a bit of a strange look, but in the end, I got what I needed, and that was what mattered.

The one problem with volunteering, of course, was that it didn't pay. As winter neared, I decided I could dip just my pinkie toe into the freelance writing world. An online local news outlet hired me to write articles about goings-on about town. I could pick and choose my assignments. This worked much better for me than the steady deadlines of *Transitions Abroad*, and the pay was higher.

A few months later, the local YMCA received a grant to help fight childhood obesity. They formed a steering committee that hired me as a publicist. I attended meetings and events, and then wrote articles about them for the local papers. The committee paid me a monthly flat fee, which meant I couldn't get tempted by working more hours than I really could. And as with volunteering with the Red Cross, the position let me focus on something health-related outside of myself, while still allowing enough time for me to make my own health my first priority.

At the start of 2009, my physical therapist Cindy said, "We're working toward skiing, you know."

I don't think I ever heard more beautiful words.

Month after month I had maintained my physical therapy schedule, until I started winning more battles than I was losing. By February, I graduated from using elastic pulleys to doing squats, abdominal exercises, and something called a "Russian deadlift." I ran grapevines along the carpeted floor like a football player. I did planks and balance exercises and pushups, until it became clear, even to the most hardcore athletes at the gym, that I was actually working out.

Still, it took me by surprise when Cindy announced that we were working toward skiing. I'd been so focused on the present that I hadn't realized an important piece of my past might be a tangible option in the not-too-distant future. "It won't be like Colorado," Cindy cautioned, "but you're definitely ready to take a run or two here in Connecticut."

I'd become such a ski snob in Colorado, swearing I'd never deign to ski on the East Coast again. Now the prospect of Mt. Southington, the little hill where I'd learned to ski as a child, glinted as attractively as the highest Colorado peak.

I hadn't skied in six years. On March 5, 2009, my dad and Janet, who had first taught me to ski, drove me to the mountain. They had planned every minute of the trip, thinking through each ounce of energy they could help save. My dad dropped me with my equipment near the lodge, then went to park the car. Janet carried my boot bag into the lodge. We chose an old wooden bench, much like the ones we'd used when I was a child, when Janet would smack the bottoms of my boots to get them on my little feet.

This time, I didn't need any help. As if no time had passed, I strapped on my knee brace, surprised that it still fit, and slipped my ski pants over it. I piled layers of thermal wear under my ski jacket, complete with a fuzzy white neck-warmer and my old, scratched helmet.

"We're only going on the bunny hill," Janet said. "You may not need all that."

"I'm going skiing." I snapped my helmet under my chin. "I'm going to dress the part. How do I look?"

"Like a skier."

When we stepped out of the lodge, I realized that the bunny hill was off to the far left. I wondered if the expense of energy skating over there would be so great that I wouldn't be able to ski afterwards.

"We could just go right to the top," Janet suggested, pointing to the chairlift in front of us that serviced the summit.

"I'm not sure I can ski that whole trail." I couldn't believe those words were coming out of my mouth, that Mt. Southington's 425-foot peak might actually be too much for me when I'd conquered 10,000+ foot mountains in Colorado. But I didn't want to mess this up. I wanted to walk away from the day feeling like I'd done it. Like I could do more.

My dad carried my skis to the bunny hill so I wouldn't have to skate, walking beside me as I slowly crunched across the snow, stopping every few steps to rest. On her skis, Janet crept along behind us. When we finally neared the lift, my dad set my skis down in front of me, the way he had so many times when I was little. He even wiped the snow off the bindings. "Ready?"

In one swift motion, I clicked into my skis. "Ready."

Skating through the lift line, left ski, right ski, felt perfectly natural. Janet and I laughed on the chairlift, knocking our skis together during the short ride. I tapped my trusty knee brace just as I once had on the chairlift in Colorado, relishing anew the feeling of the metal chair under my ski pants. When we reached the top, Janet and I raised our ski tips up, lifted the bar, and skated off the chair, just as we'd done hundreds of times before. I reached down to tighten my boots, then stopped to survey the scene. The day was sunny and unseasonably warm, like my college graduation day. I breathed in the mountain air. At 425 feet or 10,000+, it was still fresh, still invigorating. I could feel it seeping through my body, spreading healthy oxygen to my limbs.

Down at the bottom of the slope, my dad waved his arm to indicate he was ready to film. For a moment, my mind flashed to the ski day with my students at Crested Butte in Colorado when I'd had to take off my skis and walk down the slope. *What if that happens again? What if my knee gives out? What if I don't remember how to turn, or how to stop?*

"Just ski," Janet said.

And I did. My feet took over, remembering exactly what to do. Side to side they swooped, carving slow but steady arcs. I felt my thumbs pressing into my real poles, not dream poles, and smiled as the sun warmed my nose. I heard the slight breeze rustling my open pit zips and the snow shushing under my boards. I tasted the same freedom and joy I'd relished flying down the back bowls of the Rockies.

After a few turns, I stopped to rest. Janet skied up behind me. "Are you happy?"

I was crying too hard to respond.

CHAPTER 24

That summer, I returned to the scene of the crime.

Rachel and I were sitting in my apartment when she asked, "What would you think about a trip to camp?"

My first reaction was fear. Camp was the place I'd gotten sick. I couldn't possibly set foot in those woods again.

"But you wouldn't have to go in the woods," Rachel counstered. "You'd walk only on the paths, and on the beach, and of course you'd cover yourself in bug spray and do tick checks and shower every night. All the things we didn't know to do when we were counselors."

My skin tingled.

"Besides, you can get a tick bite right here in Connecticut," Rachel reminded me, waving her hand toward my patio.

My second reaction was more practical. "Camp is like five or six hours from here. I haven't gone farther than my mom's or to New York since the relapse."

Rachel waved her hand again. "I already thought that through. I'll drive. I'm thinking we go up to your mom's house after your nap one day, spend a night there, then continue on to camp in the morning and be there before nap time. Then spend two or three days up there and do it in reverse."

Eventually, my heart won out.

Rachel's in-laws had offered us their cottage down the road from camp. I was tired by the time we arrived there, but not bordering on a meltdown. As we stepped out of the car, I felt the familiar crunch of pine needles and rocks under my sneakers, heard the familiar wind rustling the trees, breathed the familiar scent of pine trees and lake air into my lungs. My body immediately relaxed, the same way it had when I'd traveled to Paris a year after my time studying there. I'd been exhausted from not sleeping on a red-eye flight, but as soon as I'd set foot in my city and smelled the pastries baking in open-air *pâtisseries* and heard the screech of the metro, my body had filled with a peace that told me, *I am home.*

After Rachel and I changed into bathing suits and doused ourselves in bug spray, we walked out the back door and down the center of a sandy path that led to a patio area and dock. The cool air was thick with fog, but I didn't care. I kicked off my shoes and ran right into the water, not even wincing at the icy chill. The lake was as clear as I remembered. I could see my feet, my pink toenails, and the rocks and sand underneath them. I was once again enveloped by the water that had swathed me for so many summers.

"You coming in?" I asked Rachel.

She shook her head. "Too cold. You can swim for me."

A small square dock was moored maybe twenty swim strokes away. I knew without questioning my capability that I could reach it. I did a few strokes of crawl, and then to conserve energy I switched to a slow, steady breaststroke, gliding long to rest, keeping the dock in my line of vision each time I came up for air. It was only a few minutes before my fingertips brushed its slimy wall.

"You did it!" Rachel shouted. "You gonna dive?"

I hoisted myself up the metal stairs and stepped to the edge of the dock. I remember how scared I'd been at age 14, standing at the edge of the five-foot diving tower at camp. Diving from that height was a requirement to achieve the swim honor I'd been working toward that summer. Every day for seven weeks I stood right on the edge, my arms against my ears, palms pressed together. I'd lean forward as far as I could without actually tipping in, my heart racing and my breathing shallow. Fellow campers who had been diving all summer, off not only that tower but the one above it that was twice as high, encouraged me from the water. I felt embarrassed and ashamed as I stood there trembling, knowing at the end of the swim hour I would walk backwards down the tower stairs and say, "Maybe tomorrow."

Toward the end of that summer my swim instructor Julia had stood behind me on the dock, tipping my body over from the waist to show me the correct form. Eventually I was so far forward that it seemed silly to stand back up and retreat. Julia sensed this and gave me the slightest push. Suddenly I was slicing through the water headfirst before I had time to think about what was happening.

"That was fun!" I exclaimed when I came up for air, hearing cheers all around. I pulled myself up on the dock, scampered up the tower's steps, and dove again. And again. And again.

On the last night of camp, counselors gave "commendations" to campers who had done something particularly noteworthy that summer. I was surprised to hear Julia say my name. Campers usually got commendations for working three summers in a row to earn the highest sailing honor, or for being particularly kind and helpful to a cabin mate. I couldn't imagine what I had done that had earned my name to be called out.

"I want to commend Jen Crystal for overcoming a major fear this summer," Julia said to the whole camp. "Jen worked all summer to dive off the tower. It took a lot of courage and dedication to climb up there every day and try, and I'm so proud of her for finally doing it and getting her swim honor."

My cheeks grew hot as the room erupted in applause. In one commendation Julia had reframed my shame and fear into courage and dedication, and suddenly instead of feeling embarrassed, I felt proud.

I thought of that commendation as I stood on the edge of Rachel's in-laws' dock. I thought about all the fear and shame and suffering that had led me to this moment. I could have looked at the "feat" of swimming a few yards to the dock as silly and easy, but only I truly knew how hard and long that journey had been.

I raised my arms and bent my knees. Then I was airborne, my feet up above my head. As I entered the water, I pointed my toes, propelled my arms so I wouldn't over-rotate, and did a little dolphin kick before bobbing to the top. I rubbed my eyes and looked toward shore.

Rachel was clapping. "You still got it!" She called out the start of a phrase coined by the camp's founder over a hundred years earlier: "Dipped in sunshine..."

Floating onto my back, I finished, "and tough as nails."

Even on a cloudy day.

That evening, we visited camp. We walked down a short, rocky path next to the dining hall that led to the lawn where everyone gathered after supper. I smiled as groups of girls wearing uniform shirts came into view. The scene was the same as it had been in 2003, the same as it had been when I was a camper, likely the same as it had been for the 100+ years that the camp had existed.

As we walked into the center of the lawn, I heard someone shriek my name. A counselor barreled toward me across the grass. When she reached me, she grabbed me in such a tight hug that I couldn't even see who she was until we pulled back. It was one of my very first campers, Jen. She used to call herself "Little Jen" and me "Big Jen." Now she was a head taller than me. "Oh my god, Big Jen, I can't believe you're here," she exclaimed. "I have so much to tell you. Guess what? I'm driving the ski boat, just like you! And look!" She reached under the collar of her shirt, pulling out her own ten-year necklace. "I got a water-skier, too! They saved the pattern from yours and used it as a stencil to make mine."

Rachel was getting her own squeals from kids she'd nannied as babies, who were now campers. She ran off to see them as I examined Little Jen's pendant. I smiled, holding out my own necklace so Little Jen could look at it closely.

She grabbed my hand. "Oh look, you're wearing your Head Counselor ring, too!"

"I never take it off," I said. "It makes me feel like camp is always with me."

"Now I need one of those," Little Jen said. "I'm still just a regular counselor. But maybe in a few years."

I remembered how badly I'd wanted to be a Head Counselor, too, and how excited I was when I was given the honor in 2001. I'd worked hard to prove my leadership in 2000, and when the invitation finally came, the satisfaction had been that much sweeter.

"One step at a time," I told Little Jen. "One step at a time."

Again, I heard my name being called, and turned to see the camp director, Pam, heading my way. As I hugged her, my mind flashed back to the summer of 2003, when we'd both been so frustrated by the ways illness had kept me from being a fully energetic leader. Now, Pam was perfectly pleasant, making small talk about how great it was that Rachel and I had made the trip, and what a fun summer it had been so far. Then she asked, "So how are you feeling?"

It was a question I heard all the time, but it seemed to carry more weight here. I wasn't sure what anyone at camp had heard about the last six years of my life, or how they might react to my actual diagnoses. I didn't blame camp for a bite that could have occurred in any woodsy area. I blamed Lyme illiteracy, which had blocked the camp nurse, me, my college Health Center nurses, and countless doctors from recognizing my rash and symptoms for what they were, just as they are missed for thousands of other patients. Still, I was concerned Pam might meet my tick-borne illnesses with the same denial that had led her to act like my mono was just laziness.

I clasped my hands behind my back and shifted from foot to foot. "Pretty good these days," I said hesitantly. "Glad to be here. It's been a tough few years."

Pam put her hands in the pockets of her faded shorts. "What did I hear you had? Lyme disease?"

"And a few co-infections."

"Co-infections?"

"Yeah, turns out, when a tick bites you, you can get lots of fun diseases, not just Lyme. They have weird names like babesiosis and ehrlichiosis."

Pam gave a hearty laugh. "Wow, those are some crazy words. What do they do to you?"

With my left foot I toed the grass. I wanted to share everything I'd learned about tick-borne illness so camp could take proper precautions. But this was our first conversation in six years, so I needed to tread carefully and slowly. I unclasped my hands and crossed my arms below my chest. "The babesiosis eats the oxygen in your red blood cells. The co-infections cause different symptoms than Lyme and can require other treatment."

"Wow. So were you just, like, in bed all that time?"

I couldn't read if Pam was judging me or offering pity. If it was the former, her opinion wouldn't have the same effect on me as it did when I was under her employ. It would, however, affect how seriously she took tick-borne illnesses, and I wanted her to really appreciate their severity so that no one else at camp would have to go through what I did just to finally be standing on this lawn again. "I was," I said slowly. "I was on an IV for almost a year and was in bed for several years before that. It was basically like having the flu and a hangover all the time."

Pam gasped. "That sounds awful."

I took a deep breath. "It doesn't have to be that bad, though. If Lyme is caught right away, it can usually be cleared up with three weeks of antibiotics. That's why it's so important for people to do tick checks and watch for symptoms."

Pam lifted her tanned, muscular arms to re-do her ponytail. "Wait, so this all goes back to that summer when you were here, and you were so sick? What did you have again then? It wasn't Lyme, was it?"

"Well, it actually was, but I didn't know it yet." I explained that in 2003 I'd had mono, and it had been so bad because of underlying tick-borne infections.

"So you really were sick that summer." The lightbulb was going off for Pam just as it had for my dad and Janet after they attended the Lyme conference, just as it often does when people have a personal reason to learn about Lyme disease.

I took another centering breath and said, "Yeah, I never should have been at camp. I didn't know how sick I really was. If I had, I wouldn't have come. It wasn't fair to anyone. Not to the campers, not to you..." I looked down.

"Or to you," Pam said.

I met her eye.

"I feel badly," she said. "I remember I was really hard on you that summer. I was always like, 'Why can't she just take a nap and she'll be better?'" She paused, then said, "I'm sorry."

"Thank you," I said. "That means a lot to me. Really, it was just that none of us knew any better at the time."

But now I did, and camp was starting to as well. A few years later Pam's mother would get a tick bite. She'd find it right away and would contact me about what to do. She'd get tested for all tick-borne diseases, and clinically evaluated. She'd be treated immediately, and she'd feel better within weeks. The camp would become very interested in learning about tick-borne illness. They'd donate to my fundraisers and ask for information to give to their nurses and staff. A few years after that, someone would send me a photo of a sign at camp that read, "Real friends check behind each other's ears for ticks!"

After waving goodbye to everyone on the lawn, Rachel and I headed down the dirt path to the camp beach. The place was deserted. All I could hear was the clink of the swim dock chain groaning against its anchor. I slid off my sneakers and socks, letting my feet sink into the cool, soft sand.

"Do you want to go peek around some of the cabins?" Rachel asked.

"Nah, I think I'll just hang out here on the beach. Why don't you come meet me here when you're done."

Rachel walked off. I stayed safely grounded on the beach. My beach. The one I'd sprinted across as a camper so I could be the first one to arrive at water-skiing. The one I'd walked purposely across as a counselor who needed to get to the ski boat. The one I'd trudged across in 2003 when the distance to the water-skiing cove felt insurmountable. The one I'd flown across in my dream with Peter, him holding my hands as we floated over a patch of blue opals.

Two years after that dream, I stood planted in place, my blue opal ring on my finger, and let my eyes do the walking. My gaze moved down the sandy strip from the swim dock to the sailboats, to the big catamaran beached by the water-skiing cove. Finally, I looked at the woods just past the cove, the entrance to the path I'd walked so many times to get to the ski boat. At this hour the woods looked especially dark next to the sandy beach. I sat down and hugged my knees, thinking about all that had transpired since I'd unknowingly crossed the line between light and dark, between safety and danger, and gotten a tick bite that had changed the rest of my life. I thought about how much damage that one tiny bug had caused.

But I couldn't fully summon anger, because when I turned my head back toward the lake, there was a magnificent sunset falling over my favorite place in the world. Speckles of sun shimmered across the waves that lapped the rocks, yellow and pink rays stretching out behind the island of trees a couple hundred yards offshore. The sky was ablaze with purples and oranges bathing Mt. Washington in the distance, sparkles dancing across the flat lake.

Absent-mindedly, I started tracing a figure eight in the sand with my right big toe, a similar pattern to the yin and yang symbol I'd made with my fingers at physical therapy. As my foot went around and around, digging deeper into darker, cooler sand, I wondered how I was to reconcile the fact that this place where I'd gotten a tick bite that had led to years of intense suffering was also the place that made me feel most alive. It was the place where I'd received the news of Peter's death, but it was also the place where I'd spent carefree nights off. It was the place where I'd gotten sick, but it was also the place that had taught me the resilience to survive that medical journey.

I stopped tracing my toe, considering disparities. So many doctors had missed the derivation of my symptoms, even though they'd tried to help me. My family had not initially understood the severity of my illness, but they had also made my life possible, and were now coming to a new appreciation of tick-borne disease. My own body had failed me at what should have been the most active time of my life, but until then it had held up through years of studying, running, and skiing. Even I had betrayed but nurtured, hated but loved myself.

I looked out at the water, at the sun sinking in the sky. Soon it would slip completely down. Even the Earth had to reconcile light and dark.

I leaned back, keeping my knees bent but extending my arms behind me and placing my palms in the sand. I tilted my head to the side, thinking. Nature held light *and* dark, not light *but* dark. Both things were true. If light and dark could co-exist in nature, then they could co-exist in me, in my body, in the people and places I loved. No one person, no one place, was all good or all bad. If Lyme, with its faulty tests and variable protocols, had taught me anything, it was that nothing is black and white. I had to allow for a gray area, for margin for error. In others, in my life, in my illness, and in myself.

I gazed at the White Mountains, watching the sun's last rays spread across the lake like golden wings. There was only a tiny margin between this moment and the sun dipping down entirely. Speckles of light sprinkled across the lake like stars just before they winked goodnight.

And I was there to catch them.

CHAPTER 25

My health remained steady through the summer, fall, and on in to 2010. I continued with freelance work. Medications, therapies, a strict sleep and nap schedule, and my specialized diet kept me humming along to a point where I was almost bored with my new life. I began to get involved with Lyme disease advocacy. Through my support group, I learned of a fundraising walk for the Tick-Borne Disease Alliance, which later became the Global Lyme Alliance. My mom, dad, Janet, Kendra, Rachel, and other friends put together a team called the Spirochete Smashers. Some of them walked slowly with me for the first loop of the 5k walk. Others continued on for me when I couldn't. I felt not only their solidarity, but that of the hundreds of other patients and caregivers there, all joined together in the fight for research and education for tick-borne illness. It was a cause I wanted to be more a part of, though I wasn't yet sure how to go about that.

In early spring 2010, I went to the library to borrow a movie that Mary had recommended. When I checked out the film, I was handed the wrong person's call slip. On it was a book called *Life Disrupted: Getting Real About Chronic Illness in Your Twenties and Thirties* by Laurie Edwards.[i] I stared at the paper as the skin on the back of my neck grew clammy. What was this book?

Life Disrupted turned out to be like a Bible for me. The author

---

i   Edwards, Laurie. *Life Disrupted: Getting Real About Chronic Illness in Your Twenties and Thirties*. New York: Walker & Company, 2008.

had a rare genetic respiratory disease called primary ciliary dyskinesia. Though we had different illnesses, her struggle for diagnosis and validation echoed my own. Like me, Laurie had been a high-functioning, high-achieving student who was sidelined by symptoms that top doctors could not pinpoint. By the time she was accurately diagnosed and treated, she had gone through physical, emotional, and mental upheaval in much the same way I had.

And she had survived to write about it.

Laurie wrote about wrestling with loss of independence; about working to get it back, and the mixed emotions that come with still needing help; about the identity crisis that comes with not being able to fulfill expectations; about navigating dating with a chronic illness. Hers was a true quest narrative. Working within the context of her illness and the limitations it imposed on her, she found a new normal. The way Laurie prioritized her needs, the way she wrote of them as just part of her forward-moving life, showed me that she didn't think of them, or herself, as a burden. They were not something to apologize for. With them, she'd attended graduate school for creative writing, gotten married, and now worked as a health journalist and college professor in Boston.

If she could do all those things with a chronic illness, maybe I could, too.

I emailed Laurie, telling her how much her book had meant to me and how I only wished I'd found it earlier. She replied that same day, saying she was excited to connect with me because she'd been searching for a Lyme patient to interview for her next book, *In the Kingdom of the Sick: A Social History of Chronic Illness in America*. She understood that Lyme was a widely misunderstood disease, and that people needed to hear about the lived experience of it. She knew Lyme patients had an underrepresented voice. Would I share mine?

On the phone, Laurie asked lots of thoughtful questions about tick-borne illness. She also told me about her graduate school program at Emerson College, where she'd written *Life Disrupted* and learned the steps to getting published. I told her about my Paris manuscript. I'd recently received a nice rejection from the big publishing house, saying that while my book was full of vivid detail and beautiful scenes, they just didn't think it would sell to a wide market. The agent, disappointed that she didn't get a quick sale, declined to send the manuscript elsewhere, so I was back to the drawing board.

"I bet you could do a lot with your manuscript at Emerson," Laurie said. "And who knows? Maybe you could start writing about Lyme disease, too, to give voice to other patients."

Hearing Laurie's story re-ignited seeds of aspiration in me. Graduate school had been my original dream when I lived in Colorado. Now that dream started to poke through the surface again. I let it emerge during quiet moments when I fantasized about my future. When I'd first moved to my apartment in Connecticut, I'd spent many evenings imagining I was in Vermont. I'd close my eyes and picture Lake Champlain. That vision remained safely tucked in my heart. I felt sure I would get back to Vermont eventually, but I began to wonder if graduate school in Boston might be the next step.

One day while Dr. O'Malley was away, I saw a different neurofeedback practitioner. She told me she often felt auras about people. I smiled politely, waiting for her to hook up my electrodes so we could get going. Then she said, "I'm getting a read of Boston from you. Do you have any connection there?"

My mom thought graduate school was a great idea because it held more flexibility than a full-time job and would likely lead to work that I would enjoy and could handle. She'd read *Life Disrupted*, and it had helped her see how someone like me had moved forward with her life. She no longer disputed my Lyme diagnosis. Instead, she wanted to help me find ways to integrate it into my life. She said, "I can picture you going to class like Laurie Edwards. I can picture you teaching like she does. I can picture you like some of the other women she describes in the book, who are sick with other illnesses." My mom's only concern was that I might become a Red Sox fan.

My dad and Janet were a harder sell. They were concerned about my ability to handle the schoolwork, about the possibility that I'd get neurologically overwhelmed in a city, and about the reality of finding medical support in Boston. Their concerns were borne of valid fears that I might land right back in the same situation I had in Vermont. Now that I was finally doing so well, they were afraid of what might happen if I rocked the boat.

To prove I could handle graduate school, I took a poetry class at a local writing center. I attended every meeting, read sample poems, critiqued classmates' work, and wrote my own. Being in a room with other writers, talking about imagery and syntax and tone, reminded me just how much I loved the craft. Ultimately, the writing class showed me and my family that Boston could very well be my next step.

My mom drove me up to do a tour of Emerson and see if I even wanted to go there, instead of jumping in sight-unseen as I had in Vermont. The "vertical campus" seemed like a good fit for my new needs. Instead of walking across a green sprawl like I had in my undergraduate days, I would take an elevator to class. I stopped by the Disability Office; they were enthusiastic about helping make graduate school work for me. After the visit, I wrote an admissions essay about my medical journey, stating that attending graduate school would shift me past surviving to the coveted step of thriving. Moreover, it would give me a chance to write a story that belonged not just to me, but to hundreds of thousands of other patients.

In spring 2011, I stalked the mailbox the way I had in spring 1996 when I was waiting to get into college. When the large envelope finally arrived, I did the same celebratory dance at age 33 that I'd done at 18. I'd been awarded a Dean's Fellowship!

I researched resources in Boston, contacting an integrative manual therapist and a neurofeedback practitioner. I talked regularly to my good friend Megan, who lived near Boston with her husband Casey. I also reconnected with college and camp friends in the area, setting up a support network before moving.

My dad and Janet took me to an Accepted Students Weekend. At a welcome reception for prospective students, I circulated the room in the same manner I would have before I lost half a decade to illness. I felt invigorated talking to other people my age who might become my classmates and friends. We all would be starting graduate school together, fresh. We all had stories to share.

I spent the rest of that weekend searching for an apartment that was near school and public transportation, not a walk-up, and close to amenities. Such a find wasn't easy to come by in pricey Boston, but finally I saw an affordable unit that was above a grocery store and around the block from a subway stop. That night we had Chinese food with Megan and Casey. I told them about the apartment we'd seen. There seemed to be a lot of green lights for a move to Boston, but given how much was at stake—my health, succeeding independently in a new city—I was nervous about whether it really was the right choice.

At the end of the meal, we opened fortune cookies. "Lucky numbers 7, 13, and 19," I read aloud from my slip of paper.

"No, read the other side," my dad said, just as Janet quipped, "Better go buy a lottery ticket."

I turned the paper over. Goosebumps crawled up my arms as I read the words. "No way." I looked up to gaze around the table. "This can't be real."

"What does it say?" Casey asked.

"You'll never believe me." I handed the paper to Casey. "Here, you read it."

Casey grinned as he read aloud, "You will move to a wonderful new home within the year."

CHAPTER 26

At the end of February 2013, during my second year at Emerson, a blizzard hit Boston. As I sat writing a paper, I watched the snow pile up on my high-rise patio. Despite living in the middle of a city, the skier in me wanted to get out. After skiing with my dad and Janet in 2009, I'd returned to Mt. Southington a couple times but hadn't skied since moving to Boston.

All three of my parents had helped me move into my Boston apartment, just as they had in Vermont, and then my mom had stayed with me for the first week. She was nervous that I wouldn't be able to manage getting groceries, doing laundry, and navigating the city without wearing myself out, but I'd done just fine. She'd stocked my freezer with meals, I'd purchased a rolling cart to take to the grocery store downstairs, and we'd found the nearest pharmacy. By the end of that first week, I was still full of vim and vigor. "I think you're going to do great in Boston," my mom had said when she hugged me goodbye.

And I had. That first summer I started appointments with my new integrative manual therapist and neurofeedback practitioner. After much research and many failed attempts at finding a Lyme Literate primary care doctor, I met one whose mother happened to have chronic Lyme disease. She understood tick-borne illness in a way that many doctors who fell in the IDSA camp of the "Lyme Wars" turned a blind eye to. My difficulty in finding her showed me just how important it was to write and share my lived experience.

My doctor's own personal experience lent her the expertise to see past the fear and denial of so many of her colleagues. She was willing to work with Dr. Raxlen; she would treat acute infections in the context of my tick-borne illnesses, and he would oversee the management of the chronic conditions.

With my medical care established, I was able to spend the rest of that summer before school just exploring and settling in. Though a cab driver told me it would take seven years for me to officially become a Bostonian, by the time I matriculated at Emerson that fall, I felt very much at home in my new city.

I loved school. I workshopped chapters of my Paris memoir *Et Voilà*, learning ways to deepen the narrative. I poured over classmates' pages that taught me about the particular difficulties women face in the military, about growing up gay and Catholic under World War II-era Italian immigrant parents, about fleeing family strife to teach English in Korea. Our experiences were different, but we shared similar doubts, questions, and hopes. Reading each other's work helped us better understand the human experience.

My classmates became trusted friends. Socializing with them brought fun back to my life, something I had literally only dreamed of when I was at my sickest. These friends hadn't known me before I was sick, nor had they known me in the darkest days, though certainly they were learning about both periods as I started writing about them. In the present, they knew a writer who had to take naps and go to bed early but was otherwise up for dinner parties and game nights. My new friends hugged me when I turned into a pumpkin at 10:00 p.m.; they threw New Year's Day instead of New Year's Eve parties; and they laughed along with me when I mixed up my words, tuned out in class, or accidentally ordered a gluten-free beer, forgetting it still had alcohol in it. One night when we met some medical students at a bar, we started talking about Lyme disease. My classmate Lauren explained to the medical students how spirochetes cross the blood-brain barrier, and the neurological damage that breach can cause. I saw narrative medicine in action that night: patient stories helping doctors understand a disease, opening lines of communication.

My classmates also saw in my story something I hadn't yet seen myself: Post Traumatic Growth. When Lauren mentioned this term to me, I thought she meant Post Traumatic Stress Disorder (PTSD). An Air Force veteran who was familiar with both trauma and reflection, she saw the latter in my writing. She told me that the theory of Post Traumatic Growth posits that beyond developing resilience, veterans and others who have experienced trauma have the ability to grow from their experiences and change their lives for the better.[i] Lauren saw that type of growth in my work, and in my life. "Your story is not just for Lyme patients," she said. "Anyone who's experienced trauma can learn from it."

One day an article appeared on boston.com that provided some misinformation about Lyme disease. I penned an op-ed in response, concluding, "I am living proof of the damage this gross illiteracy of tick-borne illness can cause. If my story can save one person the trouble of all that I have been through, the pain and suffering will have been worth it."[ii] The piece was published, and lymedisease. org then re-posted it, asking if I could write more blogs about my experience. I wrote about every aspect of living with tick-borne illness: about brain fog, about insomnia, about nightsweats and air hunger. I wrote about learning to think of my restrictions as needs. I wrote about the challenges of dependence for patients of any persistent illness. I wrote about doctors who don't listen and doctors who do, about the gender gap in diagnosing and treating illness, about the validation that all patients deserve. There was so much to share, and a thirsty audience.

As I wrote and did schoolwork, I was hyper-protective of my health, recognizing and putting out small fires before they turned into an uncontrollable blaze of relapse. I skimmed books when they were too much to read; I never missed a nap, no matter what amazing guest speaker was visiting school; and I declined invitations to events like rock concerts. I built enough margin for error into my life that the bottom was likely not going to drop out, at least not as drastically as it had in Vermont.

I waited until I successfully completed the first year of graduate school before I considered adding exercise to my routine. That summer of 2012, I took a Duck Boat tour, seeing the sights of Boston via amphibious vehicle. As we puttered across the

i   https://www.apa.org/monitor/2016/11/growth-trauma
ii   https://www.lymedisease.org/jennifer-crystal-lyme/

Charles River, the tour guide pointed out Spaulding Rehabilitation Hospital. I looked over to see people kayaking and canoeing near the hospital's dock. "They have an adaptive sports program for patients with various disabilities," our driver said.

I almost dove off the Duck Boat.

As soon as I got back to my apartment, I called Spaulding and explained my history as both a camp counselor and a patient of chronic illness. I began volunteering with the adaptive sports program one morning per week for a 90-minute session. I helped transfer wheelchair-bound athletes onto hand-powered bikes; I attached special paddles to big Hawaiian Outrigger canoes for athletes who could only use one arm; and I helped paddle those canoes. There were always six to twelve of us in the boat, so if anyone, including me, needed to stop paddling for a while, the others picked up the slack. As we floated across the Charles River, I learned the athletes' stories. Some of them had been through far worse physical adversity than I had. Some of them had experienced the same loss of independence as I had. Some of them would never get it back. But all of us were out there, enjoying our time in the sun as best we could.

That fall, as I started my second year of graduate school, I added yoga to my weekly routine, which helped me maintain the muscles and core strength I'd built over the summer. By the time the blizzard hit in February 2013, I felt ready to ski. Most of my classmates were not skiers. Just as I was thinking I'd go by myself, my friend Paige piped up, "I'll go. I'm not much of a skier, but I used to live in Colorado."

On March 1, 2013—almost four years to the day after my first foray to Mt. Southington—I texted Paige, "Here we come little Nashoba Valley! There's a 32-inch base of snow just waiting for us!"

This time I was at the wheel of the ski adventure, driving our rental car forty minutes northwest. It was a weekday, so we had the ski area to ourselves. Paige insisted on carrying my boot bag to the lodge, an act of generosity that probably bought me an extra two runs' worth of energy. I carried my skis.

We took the chairlift to the summit, a mere 422 feet in elevation. Four years earlier, going straight to Mt. Southington's 525-foot summit had seemed like too much for me. Now I felt confident and capable.

At the top, Paige said, "So, I've skied before, but it's been a while. I could use a lesson."

I clapped my mittened hands. "Well, my friend, today is your lucky day!"

I pointed to a flat area above one of the trails. "Let's glide over there to start. Use your poles to push off," I demonstrated, "and then glide from one ski to the next." Giving myself a good heave forward, I glided on my left ski, then swooshed to the right, slipping into the same rhythm I'd learned as a child, the same rhythm that had carried me across the "flats" in Colorado.

Paige shuffled along behind me, not yet finding her own rhythm but nevertheless making her way. "It's so beautiful here," she said.

I looked around at the snow-covered pines, their limbs sagging under a glistening white blanket. I felt the packed snow under my skis, breathed in the crisp air, looked out at the short run below us. It wasn't the Rockies, but Paige was right.

"Do you want to ski down first, or do you want me to?" I asked.

"Oh, you go first," Paige said quickly.

I pushed off, my skis naturally carving short arcs, my poles seemingly planting themselves without me thinking through the motion, the way I'd once been able to think in fluent French without having to translate in my head. After eight or ten turns, I slid to a stop at the side of the trail. Taking a quick sip from my water pack, I waved one of my poles at Paige. "Go for it!"

I watched her point her skis in a pizza shape and cautiously make a few wide turns. I could see that she needed help figuring out what to do with her poles. When she snowplowed to a stop next to me, she said, "I told you I'm not much of a skier."

"Of course you are!" I pointed up to the area we'd just conquered. "You just skied that whole section!"

"Any tips?"

"I noticed that you're kind of dragging your poles behind you, and that's pulling your whole body back and making you unsteady. Try holding your hands out in front, like you're carrying a tray of hot chocolate." I turned my own poles sideways and held them level in front of me. "You want to hold the tray steady, so you need to keep your arms even. If you lift or drop one of your arms, the tray will fall." I shifted on my skis. "I'm going to pretend my poles are a tray and hold them out to practice keeping my hands steady. You go down first, so you can watch me do it."

Paige skied over the next crest and then stopped to look up. Pushing off with just my skis, I made a few slow, exaggerated turns, never moving the "tray."

"Wow, I see exactly what you mean," Paige said when I stopped. "Your arms never moved. No hot chocolate would have spilled."

"Exactly! Now you try it."

I skied down a bit further so I could turn to watch Paige. She fumbled getting her poles flat in front of her, but once she did, her whole stance changed as she made turns. With her shoulders steady and her hands out in front, Paige's weight shifted from leaning back to pitching forward, and her skis naturally turned. "I'm doing it!" she shouted as she went by.

Mid-morning, we went inside for a break. We sat by the window, eating clementines. Paige pointed to a trail to the right of the one we'd been skiing. It had a mogul field on one side and a groomed section on the other. "I want to see you ski those moguls," she said.

I eyed the bumps. They did look fun, but I hadn't been in moguls since Colorado. "I don't want to get too cocky with my knee." Then I quickly added, "Well, they're not that big. I think I could do it." I was feeling so much like my old self that anything seemed possible.

Paige and I put our gear back on and rode the chairlift to the summit, where we parted ways. She skied down our usual slope, which looped around to the harder slope at the bottom, where she stopped to watch me. I took that time to survey the mogul field. I could see exactly which bumps I wanted to bounce off of, using them to help me ski a steady line. I knew my knee could handle it. I wasn't concerned about running out of steam. As soon as Paige waved her pole from the bottom, I set off.

I only skied two moguls before I chose to bail. I hadn't been able to see, from my perch at the top, that the backside of the moguls were icy, but I could certainly feel my skis scratch across them. Without a second thought, I headed right over to the groomed section, knowing that icy moguls were not a risk I needed to take. Not a show I needed to put on, anymore.

The groomed section had its own surprise. Light snow had

fallen the night before, landing in swirls on top of the smooth part of the trail. My skis ate it up. *Swish, swish, swish*, I carved tight slalom arcs one after the other after the other. I didn't stop to rest, didn't think about needing to rest. My feet were in control, and they were going to take me all the way down that slope. They were going to give me a great ride, even without the moguls.

And that was good enough.

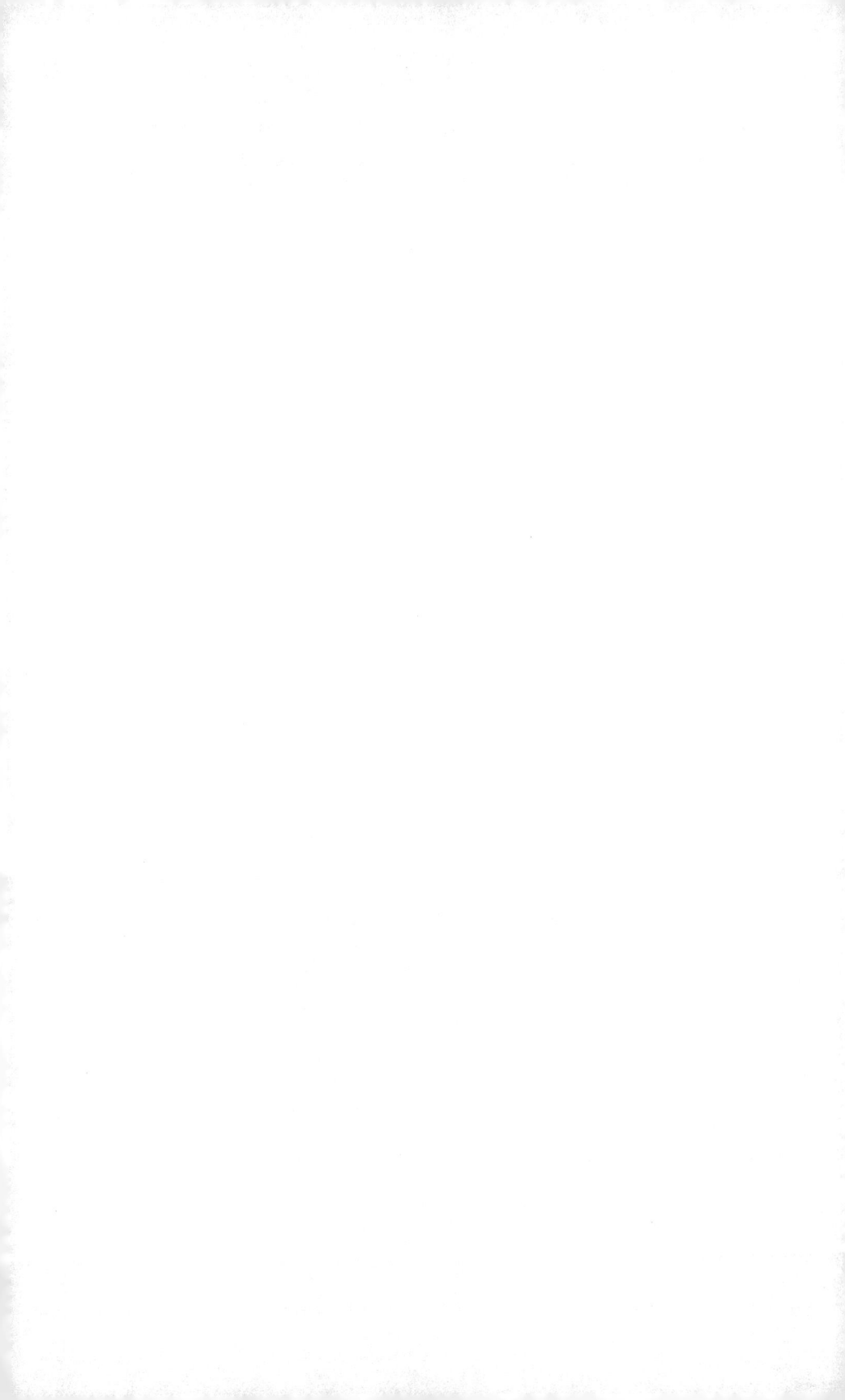

EPILOGUE

2023

One tick stopped my clock for so long. When I turned forty a few years ago, a friend pointed out that I'd been wrestling with tick-borne illness for more than half my life. That blew my mind.

Reflecting now, it's hard to believe that I've been sick for longer than I've been well. While I still straddle two worlds, especially as I now wrestle long-haul COVID-19 symptoms, these days I feel much more rooted in the kingdom of the healthy.

My new normal is different than my old normal, but I am living a full and happy life in the context of chronic illness. I've sustained that life for more than a decade, despite minor flares and other acute illnesses. I've comfortably outgrown certain limits, stretching my work, exercise, social, and travel muscles in ways I couldn't have imagined when I was bedridden and hopeless. I've seen gains I never thought possible.

After much revision in graduate school workshops, *Et Voilà: One Traveler's Journey from Foreigner to Francophile* was published by Belfort and Bastion in 2015. The road to publication, like my road to health, was much longer than expected. I had to work hard to deepen both narratives, but doing so made the successes that much sweeter.

Turtles have remained my mascot since graduating from Emerson. Now a teacher of Writing to Heal, I draw the image of that spiraling path on the board for my students, reminding them that grief or illness, like writing, do not follow a linear process.

I explain how I wanted so desperately for my own narrative to be one of restitution, but that it wasn't until I stopped trying to fit my story into that box that I truly started to heal. For me, for so many, there is no going back. When we drop the idea of our stories resolving as they "should," tying up with neat little bows, we can unwrap a beautiful gift: life outside the lines, on our own terms. Helping students come to terms with and for their own narratives, be they of illness or any other adversity, is one of the greatest gifts I've been given in my new life.

I teach Writing to Heal at Grub Street Creative Writing Center in Boston, and for five winters I also taught it as an intensive Winter Term class at my undergraduate alma mater. Yes, I finally returned to Vermont! Not in the way I had imagined, but in the way I believe I was ultimately meant to. For those winters, I got to spend the month of January successfully living, teaching, and skiing in Vermont, reconnecting in health with what my professor John Elder called "the mountains of home."

Skiing has become part of my identity again. The exhilaration I felt that day at Nashoba Valley with Paige is something that's continued to blossom. I can now ski full mornings—even two in a row!—at larger New England mountains. A friend who saw a recent video of me skiing commented, "I'd recognize those turns anywhere."

As fine-tuned as my self-care has become, I still sometimes push my body too hard and pay the price. One day I skied more runs than I really was capable of. By the time I finished the last run, I was crying, because my nervous system had become so overwhelmed by the physical exertion. I had to go straight to bed. Instead of sleeping, my body twitched and my mind spun. Moments like this scare me into thinking I'm relapsing again, but thankfully, that's never actually happened. Within a few days, I always bounce back, and I continue to monitor my needs and make every attempt not to violate them.

I can't yet imagine taking an overnight flight to my beloved Paris or traveling to the high altitude of Colorado, but that doesn't mean those dreams are out of the realm of possibility. I like to think that they, like so many others, may be achievable in time. And if they're not, that will be okay, too. Though I sometimes get frustrated by what I can't do, 95% of the time I'm amazed and humbled by what I can. A second chance at life, even an altered one, has shifted my perspective.

Peter taught me that I don't have to choose the pain anymore. I try to remember that advice when I'm confronted with choices of fear or love, anxiety or faith, self-criticism or self-care. I also try to remember that there is gray area between these extremes. Part of not choosing the pain, I've learned, is letting myself off the hook a little when I do make a bad decision. I try to choose love and joy in my life, but I am a work in progress.

Peter's mother Mary remains a good friend. After graduate school, I visited Mary and Mark in Minnesota to mark the 12th anniversary of Peter's death. Even though I'd never been to the house with Peter, I was immediately comfortable there, wrapped in his presence in a healthy way. I stayed in Peter's bedroom, leaving two pennies in the drawer of his desk, just as I'd seen two pennies left for each of us in one of my dreams. When Mary and Mark sold the house a few years later, they told me the pennies were still there, just as my dreams are still there, just as the lessons Peter taught me and the love he showed me have stayed with me as I've moved forward.

During my visit to Minnesota, Mary and I threw flower petals into the lake behind their home, where Peter water-skied and swam, where his ashes are spread. With each petal, we told a memory or thanked Peter for something. As I tossed my last petal, there was a flutter in the water, and suddenly something sprang to the surface. "Look!" Mary exclaimed. "A turtle!"

Over the past decade of burgeoning successes, there have been challenges, too, as there are for anyone. Upheaval has rattled but not broken me, because I now have the proper defenses in my body. I have a support system. Most of all, I have self-love, a gift I waited far too long to give myself.

My family's understanding of tick-borne illness, and their support, has expanded. My sisters have grown up. They have caught up and surpassed me in milestones, but now that they are adults, the age gap feels smaller. More importantly, I no longer feel tied to a prescribed timeline for life.

The friends woven into my story remain deeply ingrained in the fabric of my life. When I get over-tired and off-kilter, they are there to pull me back, to pull me up, to remind me how far I've come. The bottom has dropped out so many times in my life, but it never has with these friends; they're the people who are there to catch me when it does.

Paddy's wisdom still guides so much of what I do and what I write, but sadly it now comes from a place of memory. In 2014, he suffered a seizure and was diagnosed with stage IV glioblastoma, the same aggressive brain cancer that claimed the lives of Senators Ted Kennedy and John McCain. Though Paddy and his wife and young daughter lived in Colorado, he received treatment in Boston, so I got to see him during his two-year battle. Over meals, we discussed mortality, fears, the big questions. We always circled back to a lesson Paddy first taught me in college: the only reason we're really here is to love each other.

Paddy passed away on February 4, 2016, the day after what should have been Peter's 39th birthday. Paddy was 38. He died as he lived, with humility and grace. I was in Vermont, about to teach my final Writing to Heal class of that Winter Term, when I received the news. Earlier that shining sunny morning, I'd felt compelled to walk up the hill toward the college's chapel—the hill I'd struggled to conquer a decade earlier, the chapel that had given me strength when my faith faltered. That day in February 2016, I took a panoramic video of the chapel and the view from it of the Green Mountains. I texted the video to Paddy, reminding him of the scripture passage carved on the chapel: "The Strength of the Hills Is His Also."

The message didn't reach Paddy in time, but it did reach his family. An hour after I texted, Paddy's wife called to tell me that Paddy had died early that morning, and that she, their daughter, and Paddy's mother had watched the video as they sat around him.

A few days later, when I arrived back home, a package from the college was waiting in the mail. The only thing inside, with no note, was a screen-cleaning cloth with a printed picture of the chapel on it.

In one of our last conversations, Paddy's parting message was, "Don't let the noise and the traffic get in the way." In the depths of my relapse, he'd had me visualize slowly driving my dented Jeep out of a ditch. He'd said, "There's a rest area up ahead. Can you see it?" That rest area turned out to be a three-year layover in Connecticut, where I had to learn to acknowledge red flags so that I would not drive myself into a ditch again. I confronted roadblocks that were keeping me from truly moving forward and learned to love and trust my imperfect body. Before his passing, Paddy encouraged me to stay focused on what's really important as I, on the road once more, drive on.

I continue to try, for both of us.

ADVANCES IN UNDERSTANDING OF TICK-BORNE DISEASE

Since I started writing this book, research and support of tick-borne illness has grown, though there is still more work to be done. With an explosion in case reports, the CDC is, thankfully, beginning to change its tune on Lyme diagnosis and treatment. They have formally recognized that Lyme disease requires a clinical diagnosis, and their website now notes, "The state of the science relating to the persistent symptoms associated with Lyme disease is limited, emerging, and unsettled. Additional research is needed to better understand how to treat, manage, and support people with persistent symptoms associated with Lyme disease."[i] Though "chronic Lyme" is still a heated term, many doctors who previously denied its existence now at least acknowledge patients' suffering. Those on either side of the divide are exploring different reasons that patients might have persistent symptoms, including ongoing infection but also including inflammation, immune dysregulation, and damage to nerve pathways.[ii] These options may not be mutually exclusive, and they may not be the same for every patient.

Researchers are working hard to find answers and create better diagnostic tests, and organizations are working hard to train physicians and raise awareness. In 2016, Massachusetts legislature ordered

---

i   https://www.cdc.gov/lyme/treatment/index.html
ii   Rebman, A. W., & Aucott, J. N. (2020). Post-treatment Lyme Disease as a Model for Persistent Symptoms in Lyme Disease. *Frontiers in Medicine, 7*, 57–57. https://doi.org/10.3389/fmed.2020.00057

insurance companies to cover long-term treatment for Lyme disease[iii]; other states have followed suit. In 2017, the Department of Health and Human Services started a Tick-Borne Disease Working Group. Major medical schools like Harvard, Johns Hopkins, and Columbia have opened Lyme research and/or treatment centers. As research expands into why COVID-19 symptoms persist, my hope is that understanding of other long-haul illnesses will continue to grow as well.

---

iii   https://malegislature.gov/Laws/SessionLaws/Acts/2016/Chapter183

ACKNOWLEDGEMENTS

I started writing this memoir in graduate school in 2011. The road to publication has been long and winding. The book never would have been completed, revised, and published—nor would my health have flourished through that process—without a steady river of support.

To the mystery person who checked out Laurie Edwards' book, and the librarian who handed me the wrong call slip, you set in motion the life changes that ultimately led to me writing and publishing this book. Thank you, Laurie, for helping me see what was possible, and for leading the way. I am forever grateful to my classmates and our professors at Emerson College, who knew this book when it was only an idea and saw me through early chapters. For your encouragement and feedback, thank you to Lauren Kay Johnson, Paige Towers, Emily Avery-Miller, John Fantin, Caitlin McGill, Ashley Wells, Catie Joy, Krysta Voskowsky, Shannon DeScioli, Elliot Tetreault, Martin Hansen-Verma, Dorian Fox, Emily DaSilva, Deme Rivard, Lea McLellan, Grant Bradley, Anna Bez, Miranda Moody Miller, and Elaina DeBoard. Thanks also to Rebecca Linke for sharing one graduate school class with me, inviting me to Passover Seder, and subsequently becoming one of my best friends.

From writing workshops grew the Rest Haven Writers, who shared the entire journey of this book, believing in it and me when I lost faith in both. I raise a cheer to Kendra Ekelund and the Wales family for opening Rest Haven to us. It is a true haven for our group.

I especially could not have gotten through these last few drafts of the book, and might have given up on it entirely, without Lauren "LDogg" Johnson's encouraging Marco Polos. Thank you for virtually and literally scooping me countless bowls of ice cream over the years. If not for Paige Towers, I never would have submitted to Legacy Book Press LLC, which turned out to be the perfect home for the book. Thank you to Jodie Toohey and her team for believing in the book's potential, and thank you Kaitlea Toohey for the incredible cover design. Thanks also to fellow Legacy Book Press LLC author Ann Batchelder for sharing her experience with me.

Emerson College professors Douglas Whynott, Richard Hoffman, Joan Wickersham, and Megan Marshall taught me more lessons and had greater impact on this book than I could ever summarize here. Their wisdom (and their books, and sometimes even they themselves) carry over into my own classroom. I still have the piece of lined notebook paper on which I copied this memoir's structure that Doug had expertly outlined on his white board. Without that guidance, this book would just be a jumbled collection of anecdotes. Many thanks to my thesis advisor Morgan Baker who, working from Doug's structure, helped me to craft and shape what ultimately became an early iteration of Part I. She and other professors also offered guidance with the publication process. I also want to thank other teachers and professors along the way, from Farmington to Middlebury College to the Bread Loaf School of English, particularly Renana Kadden and Mary Ellen Bertolini for their ongoing support of both my writing and my teaching.

Nothing informs my writing more than my teaching. I have learned with and from students at Middlebury College, Lesley University, and Grub Street Creative Writing Center, as well as from one-on-one writing clients. I want to give a special shout-out to my first J-Term class at Middlebury (2015), particularly Mack Hale, D.O., who has remained a friend and a disciple of narrative medicine as he's pursued his own medical education. I also want to especially thank my Grub Street Writing to Heal students, some of whom I've worked with since 2015 and all of whom know exactly what it takes to write this type of memoir. I'm thankful for my Grub Street colleagues, especially Dariel Suarez and Chris Castellani who have patiently and generously offered expert guidance on the publication process, and who also heard my initial idea for a Writing to Heal Immersive Program and helped it come to fruition.

Thank you Sherry Schwarz for accepting my chapter for *Abroad View*, for hiring me for *Transitions Abroad*, and for being so compassionate when I relapsed. Thank you Carol Johnson for helping to facilitate my position with the Wilton YMCA, and for writing a pinch-hit graduate school recommendation. I thank *Middlebury Magazine* and boston.com for publishing my first pieces about tick-borne illness, and Dorothy Leland for re-posting the boston.com piece on lymedisease.org and then inviting me to be a guest blogger. That important step helped launch my career as a Lyme writer. I'm incredibly grateful to Global Lyme Alliance (formerly the Tick-Borne Disease Alliance) for bringing me on as their weekly columnist and giving me a platform for a decade and counting. I extend gratitude to all my colleagues at GLA over the years, most recently Lindsy Swift. Ten percent of the royalties earned from sales of this book will be donated to GLA.

I'm glad for comrades in the Lyme community like Brandi Dean and Kerry Lang, and I thank Pamela Weintraub for hiring me to write a guide on living well with chronic illness for Aeon's *Psyche*. Many thanks to other publications that have given me a voice over the years, including *The Boston Globe*, WBUR's *Cognoscenti*, and Harvard Health Blog.

Thank you to my family, especially Patti Klein, Michael and Janet Crystal, Nancy and Steve Hershcopf, Alaina Crystal and James Frankis, and Elizabeth, Reid, Jaxon, and Dylan Miller, for sticking by me, learning along with me, and making so much of my medical recovery possible. Thanks especially to Janet Crystal for now coming with me to my doctor's appointments and being a great patient advocate, particularly with insurance. Special thanks to Patti Klein for always reading with pen in hand, and for being my "Dial a Department Chair" editing and teaching lifeline even after official retirement.

To friends who are named in this book and those who are not, I believe Yeats said it best: "Think where man's glory begins and ends, and say my glory was I had such friends." I am who I am today because of you.

I would not be where I am today without my medical team, past and present, those named in the book and those who are not. I am forever indebted to you.

Last but certainly not least, I thank my readers, including friends and family, medical professionals, and patients, who have found meaning in my blogs and articles and encouraged me to keep going with the book.

Writing the acknowledgements section of a book is something writers dream of for years, pining for the day when they'll get to do so and often wondering if it'll ever come; it's a delicious little prize dangling at the finish line. Over more than a decade of writing and revising this book, I've woken up in the middle of the night to jot down names of people I wanted to someday acknowledge. Despite many scribbled lists, a fairly good memory, and a heart full of gratitude, now that this day has finally come, I'm afraid I've forgotten someone important. I'm reminded of Julia Roberts famously forgetting to thank the real-life Erin Brokovich when the actress won an Academy Award for the eponymous movie. In interviews afterwards, Roberts chided herself good-naturedly. I will do the same if you are my Erin Brockovich and ask in advance for your forgiveness. If you flowed through my river of support at any time, whether floating by at a critical juncture or swimming alongside me the whole way, know that you made a difference. Thank you.

ABOUT THE AUTHOR

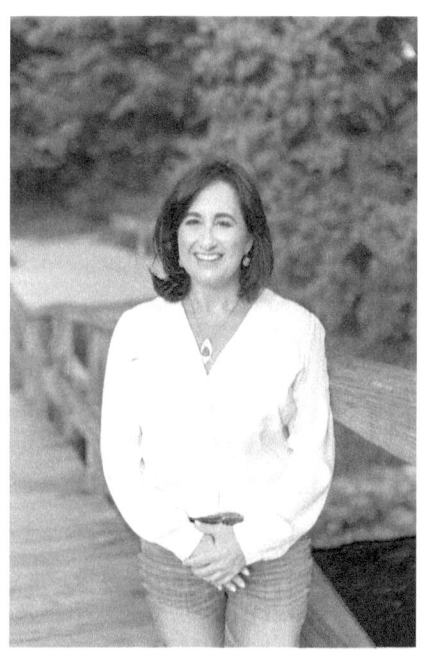

Jennifer Crystal lives and writes outside Boston, MA. Since 2013, she has been a weekly columnist for the Global Lyme Alliance (formerly the Tick-Borne Disease Alliance). The column has received mention in or on *The New Yorker*, CQ Researcher, cbs.com, weatherchannel.com, and prohealth.com. Jennifer's written work about chronic illness has also been featured in or on *The Boston Globe*, Aeon's *Psyche*, *Cognoscenti*, Harvard Health Blog, and many other publications. Her story has been featured in anthologies and articles and on news broadcasts, and she has been an invited speaker on numerous podcasts and webinars.

Jennifer teaches the Writing to Heal Immersive Program at Grub Street Creative Writing Center, where she also teaches other non-fiction courses and does one-on-one consulting. Her website is www.jennifercrystal.com.

www.ingramcontent.com/pod-product-compliance
Lightning Source LLC
Chambersburg PA
CBHW020231130626
46549CB00005B/1841